TODAY ONE GREAT DIFFERENCE BETWEEN MEN AND WOMEN IS THAT WOMEN AT LEAST *KNOW* THEY ARE OPPRESSED.

Men have heard for as long as they can remember that it is a "man's world" and that they are the privileged sex.

What they often discover too late is that their "privileges" include the right to live lives of mounting frustration, weariness and loneliness, and to die earlier than their female counterparts.

For American men are raised by parents, conditioned by society, and often encouraged by women to play a role of lover-husband-parent-breadwinner-strong-and-silent-man whose impossible demands psychically cripple and eventually physically kill them.

If you are a man, you will instantly recognize yourself and the dangers that threaten you when you read this book.

If you are a woman who loves a man, you will want both him and yourself to read it.

THE HAZARDS OF BEING MALE

"Reflects a new maturity on the part of males in response to the woman's movement . . . puts men back in touch with their emotions and their bodies and restores confidence in their proclivities."

—*Library Journal*

THE HAZARDS
OF BEING MALE

Surviving the Myth
of Masculine Privilege

With a New Foreword by the Author

by

HERB GOLDBERG, Ph.D.

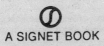

A SIGNET BOOK

SIGNET
Published by the Penguin Group
Penguin Books USA Inc., 375 Hudson Street,
New York, New York 10014, U.S.A.
Penguin Books Ltd, 27 Wrights Lane,
London W8 5TZ, England
Penguin Books Australia Ltd, Ringwood,
Victoria, Australia
Penguin Books Canada Ltd, 10 Alcorn Avenue,
Toronto, Ontario, Canada M4V 3B2
Penguin Books (N.Z.) Ltd, 182–190 Wairau Road,
Auckland 10, New Zealand

Penguin Books Ltd, Registered Offices:
Harmondsworth, Middlesex, England

Published by Signet, an imprint of Dutton Signet,
a division of Penguin Books USA Inc.

First Signet Printing, May, 1977
28 27 26 25 24 23 22 21

 REGISTERED TRADEMARK—MARCA REGISTRADA

Printed in the United States of America

Acknowledgments

There are many individuals whose assistance in the birth of this book afforded me the luxury of concentrating my energies on the more satisfying and creative aspects of writing.

First, I would like to acknowledge with deepest respect and affection my good friend, colleague, and mentor, Dr. George R. Bach. He has been a model for risk-taking, openness, positive self-assertion, and a joyous, playful, growth-oriented approach to life. Specifically, in the writing of this book, he provided many important illustrations and helped clarify critical theoretical points at times when I had reached an impasse.

I also wish to thank the many fine graduate students at California State University, Los Angeles, who were so helpful in library research and rooting out source materials. I am grateful for the fine work of Tom Maultsby whose dedication, attention to detail, skillful organizational ability, and sensitivity to the direction of this book made him someone I came to depend on greatly. Among the many other graduate students whose input was particularly valuable, I would like to express my gratitude to Donna Anderson, John Hager, Nicki Holliday, Michael Jackson, Bill Josephs, Janet Mamlet, and Jacqueline Weeks.

In addition, I am grateful to the many individuals, male and female, who allowed themselves to be interviewed by myself and my researchers—to my patients and to the patients of my colleagues whose situations and dilemmas were shared with me for the purposes of this book. While all identities and case histories have been thoroughly disguised, the struggle of the individuals for transcendence over destructive role conditioning is shared by many in our culture.

To my publisher Eric Lasher for his sensitivity, encouragement, and skill; to Marsie Scharlatt for her creative editing; to Marvin Moss for help in the practical aspects of making this book a reality; and to Lynn Cherry for her fine typing skills. My deep appreciation goes to all.

Contents

Foreword Tenth Anniversary Edition

At a book-signing event shortly after the publication of *The Hazards of Being Male* in 1976, a middle-aged couple came to the table where I was sitting, and started to look through my book. The woman commented to her husband, "This might be a good book for our fifteen-year-old son." Her husband replied sarcastically, "It'll stunt his growth," and they walked away.

A few weeks later, I went on a nationwide book tour. Men working as technicians and engineers at the radio and television stations where I was being interviewed would repeatedly ask, "Hazards of being male? I didn't know there were any." After a slight pause, I would get that kind of look men give you when they think that you're "strange." Then the inevitable question, "Would you rather be a woman?" End of conversation.

I soon learned that although I thought my book would be welcomed as a balance to the spate of negative and angry feminist interpretations of men, *Hazards* was often mocked, or simply ignored by men. Its early readers were mostly women trying to understand and relate better to the men in their lives. Many women bought it for the man they were involved with as a gift, in the hope of opening him up. Most male readers, it seemed, were those who had hit a severe crisis point in their lives and/or were reading the book at the recommendation of their psychotherapist.

I conducted workshops and gave lectures on the subject of "The Hazards of Being Male" throughout the country, and the majority of audiences were women. Men were often negative. I remember one talk in particular that I gave to a woman's organization, a chapter of AAUW. The men in the audience, mainly engineers and managers, came at the urging of their wives. They reacted with such hostility to my lecture that I thought an old-fashioned brawl would ensue.

The experiences reflected a central difference between traditional women and men: women are generally able to feel and articulate their pain, feelings, conflicts, and problems; whereas men—because of their intense externalization, the result of their traditional masculine conditioning—are out of touch with theirs. In fact, their conditioning produces a resistance to and deeper cynicism and hopelessness about change. To most men, there are no safe or viable alternatives to being the way they are. The armor of masculinity is so defensive and powerful that maintaining their self-destructive patterns of behavior and even death are more acceptable options than challenging the way they think of themselves.

A few years after its publication, *Hazards* began to develop a following, largely because of media attention, since it was the only book that described the male experience from an inner, psychological focus without blaming and accusing men of being oppressors, sexists, and chauvinist pigs. Also, it became a "male lib" book and I came to be regarded to as a spokesman for men. As a psychologist, I wrote *Hazards* as a personal survival guide for men, however, and had never thought of my work in terms of a movement.

I was ambivalent about the notion of a male liberation movement. On the one hand, I was pleased that men were starting to pay attention to the price they were paying for their roles and the conditioning they had undergone, and were finally beginning to recognize the "earth mother trap"; were able to give nodding recognition to the "wisdom of the penis"; were seeing the dilemmas of feeling guilty and inadequate in marriage; and had had their consciousness raised by the cold facts in the book. Specifically, men lived about eight years less than women, died from almost all major diseases at significantly higher rates, and as young boys suffered from autism, hyperkinesis, schizophrenia, stuttering, and behavior disturbances, leading to hospitalization at vastly higher rates. Indeed, there was nary a survival or health statistic that didn't show a disproportionately negative rate for men, not to mention the impoverished quality of most men's personal lives. Most men were effective work machines and performers, and everything else in their lives suffered.

As a practicing psychotherapist I was never fully comfortable with the idea of a men's movement because men's issues, to my mind, were personal development matters. There could be no movement for men like the women's movement because you cannot legislate men's right to feel or the right to have a male friend; nor could you march for the right not to be self-destructive, the right not to have performance anxiety, or not to feel guilty, etc.

Although a supportive social climate was crucial for the optimal development of men's personal, inner selves, it was not something one could fight about or blame anyone for. Personally, I was more interested in developing psychotherapeutic approaches, and my ambivalence about a movement stemmed from a fear of fueling fantasies that men's problems could be solved with external answers and solutions. Furthermore, when stripped of their idealistic veneers, movements tend to polarize people into the good guys, who agree with the belief system espoused, and the bad guys or pigs, who don't.

Worse still, altering the externals without transforming deeper process creates a temporary, misleading euphoric sense of a change occurring, which is inevitably followed by a worsened situation and greater despair because the unconscious motivating process gets buried more deeply than ever underneath a new defensiveness. The illusion that real change has been made—but it doesn't work—often occurs. Psychologically, when "right attitudes" are substituted for inner change, matters only get crazier because we are more out of touch than ever, and defensiveness is greater.

Nevertheless, I was delighted and fulfilled by the knowledge that many men felt that their personal life experiences had been accurately articulated in my book. Often I would be told, "You must have been following me around when you wrote that book." The secret to knowing the inner experience of so many men was simple: *although the content of men's lives gives them different external appearances, deeper unconscious masculine processes shape the internal experiences of traditionally conditioned men, making their personal or inner experiences very similar and often identical.*

A major disappointment for me after the publication of *Hazards* was the reaction of feminist women. Often I was described as a male apologist and anti-feminist. In fact, I wrote that feminism was a great boon to men because the rigid nature of masculine conditioning meant that men would *never* change unless women first tipped the balance. Furthermore, the stronger women became the less guilt-ridden, responsible, and self-destructive men could become. What failed to get through, however, was my firm and continuing belief that men and women are polar opposites, and that blame and guilt are misguided and result from a traditional, and therefore erroneous, unhelpful perspective.

I was naive about my hopes, however. I thought that after the publication of *Hazards* a dialogue with women would be welcomed and that women would be happy to learn about the inner experience of men. Since my book was often referred to as the male counterpart to Betty Friedan's *The Feminist Mystique*, I thought it would be greeted as a step toward bridging the male/female gap. That was not to occur. The unconscious polarization and defensiveness between the sexes that caused the rage and pain prevented goodwilled solutions and constructive approaches. Today, the bond between men and women in intimate relationships seems more fragile than ever.

Many good things have happened, however, since *Hazards* was published. Options for men have greatly increased. Men participate as active, involved, playful fathers today. They now have "permission" to make friends with and be close to other men; to express emotions; to expect an egalitarian sharing of material responsibility with women; and to engage in self-care activities such as yoga, meditation, and diet, or traditionally non-masculine activities without incurring knee-jerk impugning.

More focus and work need to be done, however, in transforming the deeper motor of masculinity that contributes to the disconnection and externalization that still characterize the lives of many men. I'm happy to have been involved in the process of drawing the early psychological maps, and continue to find great satisfaction in the fact that this book still serves as a source of clarity, personal self-awareness, and comfort for men as well as women.

Herb Goldberg, Ph.D.
Los Angeles, March 1987

Foreword

The male has paid a heavy price for his masculine "privilege" and power. He is out of touch with his emotions and his body. Only a new way of perceiving himself can unlock him from old, destructive patterns and enrich his life.

The humanistic growth movement and the feminist movement have both helped to create a climate that is conducive to altering rigid and harmful patterns of behavior. It is naïve, however, to believe that men will experience meaningful growth simply by piggy-backing the changes that are occurring in women's attitudes. Men need to arrive at their own realization of what is crucial to their survival and well-being.

It is my hope that this book will serve as a major step toward awakening each man to the way in which he denies and destroys himself daily. It is only then that he will fulfill himself as a total person and learn how to be a friend and partner to male and female alike.

Herb Goldberg

Los Angeles, California
July, 1975

1. In Harness
The Male Condition

Most men live in harness. Richard was one of them. Typically he had no awareness of how his male harness was choking him until his personal and professional life and his body had nearly fallen apart.

Up to that time he had experienced only occasional short bouts of depression that a drink would bring him out of. For Richard it all crashed at an early age, when he was thirty-three. He came for psychotherapy with resistance, but at the instruction of his physician. He had a bad ulcer, was losing weight, and, in spite of repeated warnings that it could kill him, he was drinking heavily.

His personal life was also in serious trouble. He had recently lost his job as a disc jockey on a major radio station because he'd been arrested for drunk driving. He had totaled his car against a tree and the newspapers had a picture of it on the front page. Shortly thereafter his wife moved out, taking with her their eight-year-old daughter. She left at the advice of friends who knew that he had become violent twice that year while drunk.

As he began to talk about himself it became clear that he had been securely fitted into his male harness early in his teens. In high school he was already quite tall and stronger than most. He was therefore urged to go out for basketball, which he did, and he got lots of attention for it.

He had a deep, resonant voice that he had carefully cultivated. He was told that he should go into radio announcing and dramatics, so he got into all the high school plays. In college he majored in theatre arts.

In his senior year in college he dated one of the most beautiful and sought-after girls in the junior class. His peer group envied him, which reassured Richard that he had a good thing going. So he married Joanna a year after graduating and took a job with a small radio station in Fresno, California. During the next ten years he played out the male role; he fathered a child and fought his way up in a very competitive profession.

It wasn't until things had fallen apart that he even let himself know that he had any feelings of his own, and in therapy he began to see why it had been so necessary to keep his feelings buried. They were confusing and frightening.

More than anything else, there was a hypersensitive concern over what others thought about him as a "man." As other suppressed feelings began to surface they surprised him. He realized how he had hated the pressures of being a college basketball player. The preoccupation with being good and winning had distorted his life in college.

Though he had been to bed with many girls before marriage and even a few afterward, he acknowledged that rarely was it a genuine turn-on for him. He liked the feeling of being able to seduce a girl but the experience itself was rarely satisfying, so he would begin the hunt for another as soon as he succeeded with one. "Some of those girls were a nightmare," he said, "I would have been much happier without them. But I was caught in the bag of proving myself and I couldn't seem to control it."

The obsessive preoccupation in high school and college with cultivating a deep, resonant "masculine" voice he realized was similar to the obsession some women have with their figures. Though he thought he had enjoyed the attention he got being on stage, he acknowledged that he had really disliked being an entertainer, or "court jester," as he put it.

When he thought about how he had gotten married he became particularly uncomfortable. "I was really bored with Joanna after the first month of dating but I couldn't admit it to myself because I thought I had a great thing going. I married her because I figured if I didn't one of the other guys would. I couldn't let that happen."

Richard had to get sick in his harness and nearly be destroyed by role-playing masculinity before he could allow himself to be a person with his own feelings, rather than just a hollow male image. Had it not been for a bleeding ulcer he might have postponed looking at himself for many years more.

Like many men, Richard had been a zombie, a daytime sleepwalker. Worse still, he had been a highly "successful" zombie, which made it so difficult for him to risk change. Our culture is saturated with successful male zombies, businessmen zombies, golf zombies, sports car zombies, playboy zombies, etc. They are playing by the rules of the male game plan. They have lost touch with, or are running away from, their feelings and awareness of themselves as people. They have confused their social masks for their essence and they are destroying themselves while fulfilling the traditional definitions of masculine-appropriate behavior. They set their life sails by these role definitions. They are the heroes, the studs, the providers, the warriors, the empire builders, the fearless ones. Their reality is always approached through these veils of gender expectations.

When something goes seriously wrong, they discover that they are shadows to themselves as well as to others. They are unknown because they have been busy manipulating and masking themselves in order to maintain and garner more status that a genuine encounter with another person would threaten them, causing them to flee or to react with extreme defensiveness.

Men evaluate each other and are evaluated by many women largely by the degree to which they approximate the ideal masculine model. Women have rightfully lashed out against being placed into a mold and being related to as a sex object. Many women have described their roles in marriage as a form of socially approved prostitution. They assert that they are selling themselves out for an unfulfilling portion of supposed security. For psychologically defensive reasons the male has not yet come to see himself as a prostitute, day in and day out, both in and out of the marriage relationship.

The male's inherent survival instincts have been stunted by the seemingly more powerful drive to maintain his masculine image. He would, for example, rather die in the battle than risk living in a different way and being called a "coward" or "not a man." He would rather die at his desk prematurely than free himself from his compulsive patterns and pursuits. As a recently published study concluded, "A surprising number of men approaching senior citizenship say they would rather die than be buried in retirement."[1]

The male in our culture is at a growth impasse. He won't move—not because he is protecting his cherished central place in the sun, but because he *can't* move. He is a cardboard Goliath precariously balanced and on the verge of toppling over if he is pushed even ever so slightly out of his well-worn path. He lacks the fluidity of the female who can readily move between the traditional definitions of male or female behavior and roles. She can be wife and mother or a business executive. She can dress in typically feminine fashion or adopt the male styles. She will be loved by having "feminine" interests such as needlework or cooking, or she will be admired for sharing with the male in his "masculine" interests. That will make her a "man's woman." She can be sexually assertive or sexually passive. Meanwhile, the male is rigidly caught in his masculine pose and, in many subtle and direct ways, he is severely punished when he steps out of it.

Unlike some of the problems of women, the problems of men are not readily changed through legislation. The male has no apparent and clearly defined targets against which he can vent his rage. Yet he is oppressed by the cultural pressures that have denied him his feelings, by the mythology of the woman and the distorted and self-destructive way he sees and relates to her, by the urgency for him to "act like a man" which blocks his ability to respond to his inner promptings both emotionally and physiologically, and by a generalized self-hate that causes him to feel comfortable only when he is functioning well in harness, not when he lives for joy and for personal growth.

The prevalent "enlightened" male's reaction to the women's liberation movement bears testimony to his inability to mobilize himself on his own behalf. He has responded to feminist assertions by donning sack cloth, sprinkling himself with ashes, and flagellating himself—accusing himself of the very things she is accusing him of. An article entitled, "You've Come a Long Way, Buddy," perhaps best illustrates the male self-hating attitude. In it, the writer said,

> The members of the men's liberation movement are . . . a kind of embarrassing vanguard, the first men anywhere on record to take a political stand based on the idea that what the women are saying is right—men are a bunch of lazy, selfish, horny, unhappy oppressors.[3]

Many other undoubtedly well-intentioned writers on the male condition have also taken a basically guilt and shame-oriented approach to the male, alternately scolding him, warning him, and preaching to him that he better change and not be a male chauvinist pig anymore. During many years of practice as a psychotherapist, I have never seen a person grow or change in a self-constructive, meaningful way when he was motivated by guilt, shame, or self-hate. That manner of approach smacks of old-time religion and degrades the male by ignoring the complexity of the binds and repressions that are his emotional heritage.

Precisely because the tenor and mood of the male liberation efforts so far have been one of self-accusation, self-hate, and a repetition of feminist assertions, I believe it is doomed to failure in its present form. It is buying the myth that the male is culturally favored—a notion that is clung to despite the fact that every critical statistic in the area of longevity, disease, suicide, crime, accidents, childhood emotional disorders, alcoholism, and drug addiction shows a disproportionately higher male rate.

Many men who join male liberation groups do so to please or impress their women or to learn how to deal with and hold onto their recently liberated wives or girl friends. Once in a male liberation group they intellectualize their feelings and reactions into lifelessness. In addition, the men tend to put each other down for thinking like "typical male chauvinists" or using words like "broad," "chick," "dike," etc. They have introjected the voices of their feminist accusers and the result is an atmosphere that is joyless, self-righteous, cautious, and lacking in a vitalizing energy. A new, more subtle kind of competitiveness pervades the atmosphere: the competition to be the least competitive and most free of the stereotyped version of male chauvinism.

The women's liberation movement did not effect its astounding impact via self-hate, guilt, or the desire to placate the male. Instead it has been energized by anger and outrage. Neither will the male change in any meaningful way until he experiences his underlying rage toward the endless, impossible binds under which he lives, the rigid definitions of his role, the endless pressure to be all things to all people, and the guilt-oriented, self-denying way he has traditionally related to women, to his feelings, and to his needs.

Because it is so heavily repressed, male rage only manifests itself indirectly and in hidden ways. Presently it is taking the form of emotional detachment, interpersonal withdrawal, and passivity in relationship to women. The male has pulled himself inward in order to deny his anger and to protect himself and others from his buried caseade of resentment and fury. Pathetic, intellectualized attempts not to be a male chauvinist pig will *never* do the job.

There is also a commonly expressed notion that men will somehow be freed as a by-product of the feminist movement. This is a comforting fantasy for the male but I see no basis for it becoming a reality. It simply disguises the fear of actively determining his own change. Indeed, by responding inertly and passively, the male will be moved, but not in a meaningful and productive direction. If there is to be a constructive change for the male he will have to chart his own way, develop his own style and experience his own anxieties, fear, and rage because *this time mommy won't do it!*

Recently, I asked a number of men to write to me about how they see their condition and what liberation would mean to them. A sense of suffocation and confusion was almost always present.

A forty-six-year-old businessman wrote: "From what do I need to be liberated? I'm too old and tired to worry about myself. I know that I'm only a high-grade mediocrity. I've come to accept a life where the dreams are now all revealed as unreality. I don't know how my role or my son's role should change. If I knew I suppose it would be in any way that would make my wife happier and less of a shrew."

A thirty-nine-year-old carpenter discussing the "joys" of working responded: "I contend that the times in which it is fun and rewarding in a healthy way have been fairly limited. Most of the time it has been a question of running in fear of failure." Referring to his relationships, he continued. "There is another aspect of women's and men's lib that I haven't experienced extensively. This is the creation of close friendships outside of the marriage. My past experiences have been stressful to the point where I am very careful to limit any such contact. What's the fear? I didn't like the sense of insecurity developed by my wife and the internal stresses that I felt. It created guilt feelings."

A fifty-seven-year-old college professor expressed it this way: "Yes, there's a need for male lib and hardly anyone writes about it the way it really is, though a few make jokes. My gut reaction, which is what you asked for, is that men—

the famous male chauvinist pigs who neglect their wives, underpay their women employees, and rule the world—are literally slaves. They're out there picking that cotton, sweating, swearing, taking lashes from the boss, working fifty hours a week to support themselves and the plantation, only then to come back to the house to do another twenty hours a week rinsing dishes, toting trash bags, writing checks, and acting as butlers at the parties. It's true of young husbands and middle-aged husbands. Young bachelors may have a nice deal for a couple of years after graduating, but I've forgotten, and I'll never again be young! Old men. Some have it sweet, some have it sour.

"Man's role—how has it affected my life? At thirty-five, I chose to emphasize family togetherness and income and neglect my profession if necessary. At fifty-seven, I see no reward for time spent with and for the family, in terms of love or appreciation. I see a thousand punishments for neglecting my profession. I'm just tired and have come close to just walking away from it and starting over; just research, publish, teach, administer, play tennis, and travel. Why haven't I? Guilt. And love. And fear of loneliness. How should the man's role in my family change? I really don't know how it can, but I'd like a lot more time to do my thing."

The most remarkable and significant aspect of the feminist movement to date has been woman's daring willingness to own up to her resistances and resentment toward her time-honored, sanctified roles of wife and even mother. The male, however, has yet to fully realize, acknowledge, and rebel against the distress and stifling aspects of many of the roles he plays—from good husband to good daddy, to good provider, to good lover, etc. Because of the inner pressure to constantly affirm his dominance and masculinity, he continues to act as if he can stand up under, fulfill, and even enjoy all the expectations placed on him no matter how contradictory and devitalizing they are.

It's time to remove the disguises of privilege and reveal the male condition for what it really is.

2. Earth Mother
Is Dead

Gary found his "earth mother" while he was still a graduate student working on his degree in hospital administration. She was already an R.N. working in the pediatric ward of the same private hospital in which he was doing his field training. "I fell in love with her when I saw how gentle she was with those kids in the ward. I was also turned on by the way she could take all those orders from the doctors and the head nurse, who happened to be a guy, without getting rebellious—if you know what I mean."

In Gary's mind, Nancy was one of the last of the feminine "good" women who really knew what it meant to *be* a woman. He made a big play for her and within three months they were living together.

She turned out to be everything he originally thought she was. While he was busy with school and had little income she gladly helped pay some of the bills. She cooked and cleaned and even supported some of his expensive hobbies like drag racing and motorcycles. Auto parts were expensive and she was glad to buy them when he was broke. He felt powerful and secretly gloated that when he was driving with her on the freeway and would suddenly get horny, he could get her to perform fellatio. He was sure that she would never do it for any other guy. He knew she didn't like it but was doing it because she loved him. He had the best of all possible worlds in her—a great homemaker and an eager sex partner and a woman who was also totally loyal and faithful.

"What more could I want?" he'd ask himself.

Eight months later she became pregnant and he married her. Because Gary was still barely making any money and had six months until graduation, Nancy worked until two weeks before she was due to give birth. They had a baby boy.

Two years later they had their second child. She continued

working at the hospital, taking off only a month after giving birth. At home she worked harder than ever—even cleaning the garage where he kept his motorcycle and racing car.

Six years into the marriage Nancy met a young doctor on her ward—a loner, somewhat of a non-conformist—who was into meditation and the occult. They began seeing each other secretly until Nancy accidentally left a note at home with her lover's name and telephone number on it. Gary found it and confronted her. She admitted to him that she was in love with another man. Gary became enraged and violent and Nancy ran out of the house.

When Nancy's boyfriend found out that she had told her husband about their relationship he became threatened and angry and he dropped her. Feeling confused, unsure of herself, and frightened, she went back to her husband; this time she was more servile than before and Gary became more autocratic than ever. He was able to take her back by rationalizing that she only had the affair because she had been under great stress and didn't really know what she was doing. However, he was going to show her that she had made the mistake of her life by fooling around. Now he really felt entitled to push her around.

Back at home, Nancy developed some serious symptoms. She wouldn't eat and she was slowly beginning to waste away and had to be admitted into a hospital in order to be fed intravenously. Then when she finally was eating again and came back home she refused to do any housework at all and began to ignore the children.

She stayed on her job as a nurse and secretly went to see her lawyer and a psychotherapist. A short time later she ordered her husband out of the house. He was shocked and couldn't believe what was happening. She had turned cold, bitter, and hateful toward him.

Still, Gary tried to hold on to his earth mother illusion of her. He continued to tell himself that she was psychiatrically ill and soon would "come back to her senses." Two months went by and she still hadn't. Instead she became more resistant, more independent.

At that point, Gary started to fall apart. He would come over to the house to see the kids and suddenly explode and get violent with her. She finally had to get a restraining order to prevent him from coming over at all. In retaliation he hired a detective to find evidence that would prove her an unfit mother. When that went nowhere he became depressed and anxiety-ridden.

He managed to convince her to go to a psychotherapist with him. When the therapist asked him why he still pursued her when she was clearly not interested in him anymore he said with bravado, "She's still the best piece of ass I've ever had. No one else could love her like I did, and she knows it. She'll be coming back."

Interestingly enough, Nancy had previously revealed to the therapist that throughout the marriage she had never enjoyed sex with Gary, had faked her responses all of the time, and had never had a single orgasm.

After two months of therapy sessions Gary gave up trying to win her back. At that point he started to improve. He saw his children on weekends and became a better father. He actually began to enjoy them, something he had never done during the marriage, because he was always so busy competing with them for Nancy's attention. Nancy became deeply involved with another man, but this time Gary accepted it and also began to date.

The phenomenon of the passive, submissive wife who suddenly and inexplicably turns around and leaves her shocked husband has become very common. Humiliating themselves by going to extremes to win back a woman who had rejected them, many successful, seemingly strong, self-contained, "independent" men have been brought to their knees. Men who appeared to have everything became seriously depressed and suicidal, experienced night terrors, and became physically abusive toward the errant spouse or her boyfriend. They undertook incredibly childish and degrading manipulations in an attempt to win back "their" woman.

A forty-nine-year-old patient who was separated from his wife was willingly supporting her and their child while she lived with the boyfriend she had run away with. By being a "nice guy" he hoped that she would return eventually. Where he once had been total master in the relationship he now had become total slave. She told him when he could be with their child, when they could get together, and how he would have to change for her to even consider resuming the relationship with him.

It is also common for men who have been abandoned by their earth mother to continue to believe that she wouldn't dream of going to bed with another man. "I know her like a book," is what they so often say. Invariably however, it turns out they are deluding themselves.

This abandonment by earth mother is often sudden and unexpected. It gives ample evidence of how little these men knew about their wives' or girl friends' inner feelings, believing all along that everything, including the sex, was great.

In an article published in the *New York Times* titled "I Am One Man, Hurt," the husband, a writer and public relations executive, wrote about his experience of abandonment by his wife. "I thought we were a perfectly happy family until my wife told me, without any advance warning, that she didn't love me anymore and wanted a divorce. Not a matter of infidelity or alcoholism or beating or arguments or desertion, but that it didn't mean anything to her anymore and she wanted out."[1]

A young man interviewed by one of my research assistants described it this way: "It happened with virtually no warning. I came home one day and she was gone. Then I got this letter from her saying, 'There's no point talking about it. I've made up my mind.' I didn't know if it was something I said or did or did not say or do. She felt that I should know exactly why she left. But I was oblivious to all of it. She never gave me a chance to change anything. She never even pointed out any problems. It's taken me four years to free myself from the hold—the influence she had on me. I still haven't gotten over her completely."

In all of these instances the male in the relationship collapsed—as if his energy source, his reason for living had been taken away from him. And each of these men went through a period of saying, "Without her life is not worth living."

These examples are not extraordinary or even unique. Nor were the men involved sick or atypical personalities. The phenomenon of the collapse of the male when he is suddenly abandoned by his earth mother, his supposedly "totally devoted, submissive" woman is becoming increasingly common.

The phenomenon recently was partially documented in a book that explored trends in contemporary male-female relationships. One such trend clearly emerged from the author's research. ". . . The long suffering female is largely a thing of the past. Statistics show that it is often she, and at some stages in the marriage, more often she, who institutes proceedings for divorce."[2]

According to a widespread cultural myth, the female is the more dependent one in the man-woman relationship. The male is said to be emotionally shallow and unable to maintain a deeply intimate emotional relationship with a woman. Clinical experience, however, suggests that this "shallowness" is simply a self-protective device used by the male to avoid revealing his vulnerability. That is, the male resists closeness and dependency on the female *because once the unconscious defense is penetrated by a woman he becomes profoundly attached to the point of deep and almost total dependency.* Particularly in first marriages, many males unconsciously seek a relationship of primitive dependency such as they had with their mothers, and like the baby from whom the breast is unexpectedly removed, they rage and despair when this source of comfort is withdrawn.

Recent studies on mental illness, suicide, and death seem to corroborate the theory of profound male dependency on the female and his vulnerability without her. Researchers, analyzing numerous studies on the divorced and widowed, concluded: ". . . When we compare single men with single women, divorced men with divorced women, and widowed men with widowed women, in each case it is men who are much more likely to be residents of mental hospitals."[3]

Data from the National Vital Statistics System indicates that the divorced male has an annual death rate that is more than three times as high as the divorced female.[4] In one study, researchers found that death, particularly from coronary artery disease, occurred in a group of widowers at 40 per cent above their expected death rates during the six months following the deaths of their wives.[5] A recent study on suicide revealed that in some areas of America, bachelors have a suicide rate which is more than four times as high as spinsters.[6] Still another study indicated that men who had recently lost their mothers were significantly more prone to committing suicide than non-bereaved males.[7] And recent research on remarriage indicated that the divorced male tends to remarry sooner after his first divorce than the divorced female.[8]

So it goes right down the line. The evidence strongly suggests that the man who loses his female attachment, be he divorced or widowed, and the single man who had no female attachment, are all significantly more vulnerable to mental illness, suicide, and death than the woman in a similar situation.

I have a personal pet theory, which ties in with this data, about why women in our culture live so much longer than men. I believe that unconsciously the male is afraid that he can't survive without the woman. Outside of his strong attachment to his woman, he is often an isolated, alienated being. He has few close male friends. He has suppressed his interest in other women and has been a passive, noninvolved father to his children. All his needs are invested in her. However, after a woman loses her man, she still has close relationships to nourish her, other women, and her children. Being less dependent on the male, she can make it with or without another man.

The male is deeply dependent on the female from conception on. The roots and explanations for this lie in early social and emotional conditioning. As an embryo and fetus he is placenta-dependent. At birth he is breast-dependent, and throughout his early boyhood he is profoundly dependent on his mother as his primary human relationship. *She* is the one who holds, rocks, cleans, comforts, and clothes him. *She* sets his limits, teaches him right from wrong, reinforces him with praise and controls him with punishment. The female child has also been dependent on her mother, a female figure, but has no comparable deep-rooted dependency on the male for her psychic nourishment.

Despite the bravado and noises he makes about not allowing a woman to control or dominate him in order that he might maintain his fantasy of being stronger and totally in control of the relationship, the male unconsciously comes to see the female as his lifeline—his connection to survival and his energy source. Many adult men, once they have established a primary relationship with a woman, begin to abandon almost all of their other relationships. The dependency becomes increasingly intense and the crisis, if and when she does leave him, is often life-shattering.

The female does not develop this kind of intense dependency on the male. The male was never her lifeline; she had no deep-rooted dependency on him for psychic nourishment. As a girl she was dependent on her mother and not her father. Consequently, a divorce, widowhood, or rejection by a man may be traumatic, but the trauma is a less profound or primitive one, and she can recover more rapidly.

The earth mother fantasy was also encouraged by the male's self-hatred. As a boy, nursery rhymes told him that he was made of "frogs 'n snails 'n puppy dog tails" while she was "sugar 'n spice 'n everything nice. He came to believe that she gave life and nourished it, while he destroyed it. Ashley Montagu put it this way: "Woman is the creator and fosterer of life; man has been the mechanizer and destroyer of life . . . Women love the human race; men are on the whole hostile to it."⁹ The male identified with this negative masculine image and it was remarkable to him that she was able to love him in spite of the fact that he was brutish, lecherous, aggressive—in a word, "evil." The male fantasy of his earth mother's purity was equivalent to the child's naïve belief that his parents never have sex or do dishonest things.

What is happening to the female today? Is she becoming a different person? The answer is "no." She is simply emerging, revealing her true identity, and allowing her long-suppressed aggression to surface. Traditionally, the woman felt compelled to collude with the male fantasy of her as fragile, helpless, and dependent. The male expected little more from his woman other than that she supported his self-image of strength by living up to his expectation of her as pure, loyal, passive, unfathomable, non-sexual (except perhaps toward him)—someone who supposedly fulfilled herself simply by being devoted to him and his children. She seemed quite willing to play this role of supportive, facilitating bed-rock. She was satisfied to bask in her man's achievements. He could please her simply by becoming a success and her identification was drawn from this. She was willing to play Madonna earth mother—modest, pure, sexless, and unworldly. Two psychologists recently writing on the subject put it this way:

> The typical woman . . . in courtship . . . assumed the passive, submissive, conventional, female role; in a phrase, she bolstered his ego at the expense of her own. If she was not completely swept off her feet by physical attraction, she made a shrewd assessment of his potential as a breadwinner and a bed partner, and then set about proving to him that she was what he wanted as a housewife, help-mate, and mother of his children . . . [she] . . . pretended to be more "feminine" than she perhaps really was. . . .¹⁰

Women are also denying that they fulfill themselves by playing the role of mother to their husband's children. One mother who had given up custody of her children to their father began to recognize previous emotionally unauthentic attempts to be earth mother after she was out on her own. Originally, she had wanted seven children. Now, discussing visits to her children, she stated: ". . . I realized I was seeing them out of guilt, just like I'd been living with them all those years out of guilt. It astounded me when I discovered I wasn't all that attached to them. . . . Now I'm kind of doing what men do. The children are no longer a major part of my life, in terms of the time I spend with them."[11]

(As far back as 1923, Ruth Read of Columbia University published an article in which she interviewed eighty-seven pregnant women. She asked them if they were happily anticipating their babies. Seventy-five per cent of them said "no," and gave many different reasons. Of those who answered "yes," a number did so only because their religion deemed motherhood a duty.[12] Over fifty years ago!)

Traditionally, men did not recognize the existence of female aggression. They needed to maintain an image of her as weak in order that they could deny their own dependency needs and see themselves as strong. Because women's aggression was largely repressed, it emerged in a different form from men's and reinforced the fantasy. A first-grade teacher discussed this difference as it appeared at an early age: ". . . Boys were more physically aggressive than girls, but . . . they were like 'teddy bears.' Their behavior was fairly direct and active. In contrast . . . the girls who were aggressive tended to be 'mean and devious.' "[13]

When long-suppressed female aggression finally emerges openly and directly it can take extreme forms. This was recently discussed by columnist Shana Alexander. Explaining why she abandoned her administrative role in the National Women's Political Caucus, she wrote:

> . . . the savage infighting among the feminist leadership wore me down. . . . The reason women are such crude, brutal and destructive combatants, I later decided—the reason women fighters lack pace, grace, rhythm and mercy—is certainly not because we are subject to raging hormonal impulses as some men claim. . . . I think that hair-trigger female

fury, the surge to leap for the jugular at the merest drop of a glove, the readiness to "drop the bomb on Luxembourg," results from the lack of a female tradition of chivalry.[16]

Women across the nation have begun to experience and spit out their repressed anger regarding their old role. This situation is an ego shock to many men. His façade of greater strength is collapsing. Like the nation's original reaction of disbelief to the energy crisis, the male is also having difficulty comprehending that his once seemingly endless supply of energy is drying up. He is being cut loose and pushed into an autonomy he really isn't prepared for. With all their eggs in one emotional basket some men have no wells of nourishment from which to draw. Women, however, are in a much sturdier position. They are discovering the emotional truth that they can do without men very well. They are less fearful of openness and closeness with their female peers and are able to accept and give support to one another. The male has isolated and alienated himself from other men supposedly to bring his woman the spoils of competitive victory. Now his woman also is proclaiming herself his competitor, even potentially his enemy as she harangues him with epithets of "male chauvinist pig." Not only has he lost his earth mother, but in his fear and confusion he is scrambling to be liberated, not necessarily for his own benefit, but rather to please *her*.

While women have been quite free in expressing anger toward men, men are largerly unable to express their anger toward women, particularly their resentment over loss of control in their relationships with women. In my work in aggression training, I frequently do a ritual we call the "gender club" in which I encourage men and women, single and/or married, to spew out in turn their innermost hostile feelings toward the opposite sex. Invariably, I've found that the supposedly aggression-phobic and passive female is able to do this quite readily, while the male is very blocked in his expression of anger toward women. It is "unmanly" to acknowledge openly his vulnerability or his anger. Frequently it ties in with the fear of being a bully, and consequently his anger over the situation emerges only indirectly. He becomes machine-like. He expresses anger primarily by emotional withdrawal from her, as well as from himself. He detaches himself from his rage and becomes invulnerable.

Male rage is being intensified by unconscious and conscious recognition that the old roles are no longer operative, and they may be the only roles he really knows how to play. He knows she is discovering that she is just as strong, if not stronger than he, and can survive without him much more easily than he without her. In his self-hating fantasies he may even feel that he may eventually be discarded by her completely. After all, she is now rebelling against any inference that there is such a thing as "feminine" or "maternal" behavior. Someday she may not even need him for procreation; she may even be inseminated artificially.

The male has yet to realize, however, the powerfully beneficial aspects of the female's emergence as an openly assertive, aggressive being. The earth mother fantasy is dead. The female is getting in touch with her aggression, her rage, and her strength. As one woman stated, "What we found was that consciousness-raising clarified for us what we wanted to be—valiant, independent, creative, warm, loving, assertive people—and what we wanted to have—work that was meaningful and relationships that were mutual, nurturant, sexual and non-masochistic."[13] This is the time for *his* rebirth as a total person and *his* reentry into full emotional reality. He can let go of his fantasy image of her as fragile, dependent, and pure and his perception of himself as ever-strong, independent, and evil.

By the female rejecting her role of passive reactor the male now can release himself more readily from the chronic guilt which comes from being the person who *acts* while she simply *reacts*. Sexuality is an excellent example of this. In the past the woman had denied her sexuality. Sex was supposedly *his* need, not *hers*. She took no responsibility for her sexuality so that he often was left feeling degraded and selfish for acknowledging his needs. She could also wait for him to lust and to cheat and then point an accusing finger. She was "clean" and he was "dirty." Now, however, that she is owning up to her own sexual needs this picture is changing radically.

It is informative and often quite surprising to men to hear what women are really thinking and feeling about sex. It is often in stark contrast to what men believe their earth mothers are experiencing. A ritual I often use in marathon therapy groups is called the "fishbowl." As their part of this ritual the women sit in a circle and discuss among themselves their experiences and feelings about men in bed, speaking as if the men were not present. The men sit on the outside and listen. Here are some of the comments of the women: "I wish they wouldn't worry so much about my damn orgasms."——"I'm so afraid of damaging their egos by telling them what I really want."——"Sometimes I feel like making loud noises but I'm afraid they might freak. Men are so quiet in bed."——"If I tell them I want sex or make the first move most guys freeze up. I guess they think I'm a nymphomaniac."——"Most guys feel they have to take a lot of time, all of the time. They don't seem to understand that sometimes I just want to screw and not 'make love' too. I love quickies sometimes."——"Most guys think that because we've had sex I'll expect a relationship, so they run away. Sometimes I also just want a purely physical relationship with no emotional strings attached."—— "We're supposed to be the ones who feel guilty the morning after but I think that more guys have bad feelings about it afterward. It's like they don't want to remember what they did the night before."

Most important, the male is now being released from the feelings of having to take responsibility for the woman. She is becoming an openly assertive person rather than one who unconsciously or consciously controls and manipulates him by being "helpless," or "fragile," or developing psychological or psychosomatic symptoms because she cannot express her aggression or sexuality openly or directly.

In this process of rebirth of female *and* male he can let go of his distorted perception of her and allow her to assume equal responsibility for the problems and tragedies of life. No longer need his overt and covert competitiveness and even violence toward other men be justified as necessary for the survival of his wife and family. By investing her with fragility and helplessness he took on the dirty aspects of competition and the ugliness of war. That was always man's business. He fought to prove his worthiness as a protector and provider. He can now abandon that self-destructive posture.

The death of the earth mother fantasy means that he now can free himself finally and totally from his macho pose. He can guiltlessly give *himself* and *his* needs priority, just as she is beginning to own up to hers. As she expressed antipathy toward many aspects of her role, he can also acknowledge his true feelings about the many self-denying aspects of being the diligent provider, faithful husband, dutiful father, and all-around strong man.

He'll be forced to grow in order to survive in another important way. The fantasy of the woman as mind-reader had permitted him to cling to the infantile desire to be divined, to have his needs magically recognized and met by his all-knowing, all-loving woman, without his even having to ask. He will now have to learn to recognize and acknowledge his needs and then ask for and even demand satisfaction directly and openly, or else he will experience emotional starvation. Because, in the past, he was unable to ask for satisfaction directly, he lived in hidden anger when his needs were not divined.

The man who continues to hold on to or search for the few supposedly remaining earth mothers around—women willing to play the role of the old-fashioned, selfless, passive, and devoted female—are courting emotional disaster. That is, even if he believes that he has found the only "real woman" left in the world, he is probably deluding himself. Earth mother may never have existed in the first place. Rather, it may have been a female accommodation to his need to see himself as her defender and protector, born in part, out of her fear and doubt about her ability to survive as an independent being. It was an emotionally unauthentic posture that camouflaged the full extent of her strength and independence.

Therefore, the male who thinks he has found an earth mother will only get hooked into relating to her regressively—aborting his own growth and being much less of a human being than he is potentially. He will be guilt-ridden and infantile and demand nourishment and energy from "mommy" in return for playing out his self-destructive macho role. He still will get her aggression, only he'll get it in the old indirect forms of fatigue, frigidity, depression, headaches, forgetfulness, etc. Meanwhile, he'll destroy himself playing hero-warrior-macho while alienating himself from other men in the process.

Men who already have been able to surmount stereotyped role casting and expectations and have been able to relate to the woman as an equal partner and help-mate, a person from whom they can accept constructive support as well as give it on a mutual, authentic basis, can achieve the ultimate in the man-woman relationship. For it is with her that he can potentially experience many of the deepest forms of ecstatic and fulfilling human interaction. However, refusing to see her as she is—not fragile but strong, not dependent but autonomous, not passive but aggressive, not in need of protection but a canny fighter in her own right, and not self-denying but self-serving just like himself—will lay the foundation for experiencing the deepest levels of anguish and despair.

Earth mother is dead and now macho can die as well. The man can come alive as a full person. No longer need he play powerful, successful "big daddy." No longer need he indulge in humiliating double standards and hide his unique maleness. No longer is he responsible for her feelings of fulfillment and well-being. When she is she in her genuine, total, strong femaleness and personhood and he is he in his total maleness and personhood they can begin to revel in the realities and joys of an authentic, interdependent, and genuinely fulfilling interaction.

How To Recognize The Earth Mother Trap

1. You feel alternately sentimental about her, then bored, suffocated or engulfed.
2. You feel guilty about depriving her and not giving enough of yourself.
3. You believe that you're working and doing the things you do primarily for her.
4. You believe that she's a more giving and more selfless person than you.
5. You're sure that she has no sexual fantasies or desires toward other men.
6. You feel guilty whenever you're having a good time that doesn't include her.
7. You kiss her on the forehead in fatherly fashion rather than on the lips, in a more sensual way.
8. You are exhilarated when you see her cooking for you or smell the clean laundry.
9. You feel you have to hide your sexual fantasies about other women from her because she'll be "deeply hurt" and "shocked."
10. You're sentimental about what a "good" woman she is

and how lucky you are to have her standing behind you.

11. You're glad that she's not one of those "women's libbers."

12. You're amazed at how in tune she is with you—she always wants to have sex when you do, she likes the exact same vacation places, and enjoys the same kinds of activities. Everything you like she seems to like.

13. You like the quiet life with her apart from other people, because with her as a friend you don't need any other people to be close to.

14. You need her in order to feel that you're a man.

15. You're amazed that she loves you in spite of your faults and the other terrible things about you.

3. The Wisdom
Of The Penis

... he who can sleep with a woman and does not, commits
a great sin. My boy, if a woman calls you to share her bed
and you don't go, your soul will be destroyed! That woman
will sigh before God on judgment day, and that woman's
sigh, whoever you may be and whatever your fine deeds, will
cast you into hell![1]

—Nikos Kazantzakis
Zorba The Greek

The essence and ultimate joy of male sexuality lies in the experience of total arousal, the moment when nothing in the
world exists except the woman beside him, his penis rock-hard
and going nowhere, certainly not down until it has penetrated—desire at such a peak that no fantasies could possibly
intrude and with the entry sending ecstatic waves and shivers
through his entire being.

Every man deserves that kind of sexual experience. Indeed,
it is a state most men have experienced at some time in their
lives *before* they allowed their sexual spontaneity to be mired
in intellectualizations about "sexuality," derailed by abstrac-
tions about "meaningful relationships" and "sharing," alienated from their own experience by a destructive emphasis
on techniques, and numbed by scientific teachings about the
physiology of the woman and himself. That, to my mind, is
the essence of much of the so-called new sexual enlighten-
ment—the "progress" and the problem.

While women's sexuality has been misunderstood and
they've been confused and degraded by psychoanalytic interpretations such as "penis envy," "anatomy is destiny," and
"frigidity," men, I believe, have been seriously and negatively
affected by such labels as "latent homosexuality," "fear of
intimacy," "mother fixation," "repressed hostility toward

22

women," "fear of failure," "compensation for feelings of sexual inadequacy," "castration anxiety," and "impotence."

Undoubtedly these all contain a basis in truth, but instead of facilitating his growth, the major *impact* of these concepts and terms have been to propel the male into greater self-consciousness, guilt, and self-accusatory reactions. Belief in these ideas often causes him to distrust his own unique sexual responses.

The beginning of a new male consciousness in the area of sexuality will first require, along with being fully aware of his feelings, a different way of interpreting his responses. It will demand an awareness of the constant, countless, subtle ways he has allowed himself to become conditioned into accepting the burden of sexual performance. Therefore, I will not discuss techniques or physiology here, but rather the issues and attitudes which underly the prevailing orientation toward male sexuality. Techniques are merely "frosting on the cake" primarily useful, if at all, to those who already have a spontaneous, happy sexual flow. The preoccupation with techniques commonly seen today usually signals an underlying awareness of the death of passion and spontaneity. Rather than owning up to that fact, men try to manipulate themselves back into arousal through the use of techniques. The most exotic of them are useless if the feeling is not there. The emphasis on the facts of physiology may be interesting and intellectually enlightening but has nothing to do with the *experience* of sex itself.

It is crucial to put into realistic and proper perspective the longstanding notion that the culture favors men when it comes to sex and to reexamine the myth that they are more "free." It is true that a boy is given more exploratory privileges and has traditionally been allowed a wider latitude in terms of sexual indulgence. However, cultural evaluations of his sexual behavior have been far more harsh.

Impotence

Men have been put on the defensive and often torture themselves with anxiety about so-called impotence. In our culture the subject has become an almost maniacal preoccupation.

Some writers have termed impotence a contemporary male plague. While lip-service is paid to the fact that impotence is a two-way problem, it is the male who is in the majority at the sex therapy clinics. The image of the female's role in male impotence is still largely one of helper—a sometimes supportive, sometimes resentful spectator waiting for him to overcome *his* problem.

Writers in the field of mental health often inform wives on how to help their impotent partners. One such recent, highly successful article (it was reprinted for mass distribution after being published in one of the most widely read magazines in America) was titled, "Impotence: What Every Woman Should Know." The writer, a practicing psychologist and psychotherapist, concluded as follows:

> The more experience I acquire in treating men with potency problems, the more convinced I become that a loving and concerned woman is a man's most important asset in restoring—or maintaining—his sexual capacity. When a husband's belief in his masculinity becomes eclipsed by anxiety and worry, his wife's faith and help can turn a potential nightmare into a period of renewed growth and understanding.[2]

This is a typical example of the female being cast in the role of a benevolent spectator.

Even the word "impotence" reflects the underlying attitude that exists. The meaning of the word is "lack of power." This definition itself immediately places the male on the defensive. His self-image demands that he do anything not to seem powerless.

Performance fears, achievement fears, and competition fears are often credited with responsibility for male potency problems. In "A Clinical Study of 'Coital Anxiety' in Male Potency Disorders," the following fears were listed: 1) fear of failure, 2) fear of ridicule, 3) anxiety over the size of the genitals, and 4) fear of detection.[3]

The emphasis on male "fears" as being the problem in impotence subtly places the responsibility directly on his shoulders. It is saying, "If you could only overcome your fears then you would be all right as a sex partner."

The psychoanalytic and psychiatric approach to impotence, which involves tracing back and exploring early experiences and traumas, has a basis in reality but is a little like treating food poisoning by exploring early eating habits. It neglects the fact that the real cause may be in the present, with the body appropriately responding to something that it seeks to avoid.

I therefore would first translate the ugly language of impotence into its non-intellectualized, gut-level meanings. So-called primary impotence, which means *never* being able to get an erection, is considered extremely rare and will not be considered here. The vast majority of men *are* of course capable of becoming erect under certain conditions and with certain women. So-called impotence is almost always a pair-specific phenomenon, that may be making a powerful statement about the man's feelings about the relationship toward the particular woman he is in bed with. Ironic as it may seem, most men, would rather feel they have a medical problem than say very simply to their intimate, "I don't want to make love to you." In other words, acknowledging impotence and claiming, "I've got a problem," is easier than expressing the feeling, "I'm not turned on by you." Therefore, instead of seeing himself as impotent, I would encourage him to say "I don't want to have sex with you." I would have him translate "premature ejaculation" into, "I want to get this over with as fast as possible." I would encourage him to explore and understand his negative responses to the particular woman or situation rather than assume the burden and then try to overcome the "symptom."

My clinical experience indicates that the man who diagnoses himself as impotent is often experiencing something within his relationship or about his partner that is killing his desire. However, the feeling message is only being telegraphed by his body response and is not being recognized in his conscious brain.

A colleague of mine is treating a forty-one-year-old man who became impotent after he lost his job. The patient previously was informed by one well-meaning doctor and had also read in several magazine articles that his inability to achieve erection had something to do with the fact that he associated his job with his masculinity and the recent loss of his job was a threat to his ego. Therefore, because he was no longer able to feel dominant and "like a man," he was also unable to function sexually. The explanation sounded reasonable enough, but it didn't help this man.

An in-depth interview with his wife revealed that she was secretly deeply resentful about his unemployment and blamed him for his lack of foresight. Out of guilt, however, she never told him, but she did say to the therapist, "He knew it was bound to happen and he could have done something about it in time, if he had really wanted to." The man's penis was perceiving her unspoken anger and her attitude of rejection toward him and was refusing to "make love" in the face of her anger and rage.

Here's another situation in which penis wisdom was more perceptive than conscious thought. A wealthy and successful divorced man in his early fifties came to therapy in a panic because he couldn't get an erection with a number of his young girl friends. He wondered if he was getting too old. In the process of talking about his "problem," he began to realize that the young women he was involving himself with were relating to him as a symbol of success and were attracted to his wealth, rather than loving him as a person. It made him feel isolated and used. He knew that if he didn't spend large sums of money on his girl friends they would rapidly lose interest in him. His non-responsive penis was sounding the alarm and protecting him from getting deeply involved in a relationship that would be loveless and manipulative, a relationship in which he would only be used.

A different form of the wisdom of the penis is illustrated by the responses of a twenty-six-year-old recently married engineer. He came to therapy in a severely anxious state because he was ejaculating prematurely and his wife was castigating him for this. The twenty-nine-year-old wife had had two years of psychology courses and had convinced him that he was really angry toward women because of the way his mother had treated him. She said that he was reacting to her like a mother and was punishing her by not satisfying her sexually. That sounded plausible to him and he came to therapy wanting to be "cured." Several private sessions with his wife, however, brought to light the fact that she had married him primarily because she was approaching thirty and was concerned that she'd never get married. She revealed that she had never been attracted to him physically and had been faking her sexual excitement right from the beginning. She continued, "I do everything to make him think he's a real tiger!" His penis was aware of her basic lack of true involvement with him. His premature ejaculation could be interpreted as not wanting to make sustained contact with her and discover that she had no genuine sexual and loving feelings for him.

An associate of mine told me of a patient who had recently gone to bed with the wife of a friend of his and found himself impotent. As he explored his reaction he realized that she probably was only using him to precipitate an end to her own faltering marriage. His body sensed this and wisely kept him out of a potentially explosive and dangerous relationship.

In another instance, a forty-two-year-old man became completely impotent with his wife of seventeen years. However, he was extremely potent during occasional visits to prostitutes. When I first spoke to him he was in an extreme anxiety state regarding his inability to perform sexually. He wanted to be "cured" as quickly as possible. He even asked to be put under hypnosis in hopes that I could suggest his erection back.

As we spoke at greater length however, it readily became apparent that internally he had been experiencing rage toward his wife for many years. In fact, he admitted that he had been using fantasy imagery of other women all those years to arouse himself with his wife. He had been having no spontaneous sexual response to her at all. Recently, the imagery stopped working for him and he could not get an erection with her under any condition.

He acknowledged that he felt smothered and engulfed by his wife whom he felt resented him and tried to block his every autonomous move. He had been unable to assert himself with her. Instead he had given up his own activities—like going out for a drink or golfing with friends, playing cards on a weekday night, or going on a monthly fishing trip. He simply went to work and came home.

While consciously he rationalized his wife's demands and stated that he felt she was justified in her expectations and requests to have him at home with the children, his penis registered his innermost feelings. It was protesting the annihilation of his real self. It was his "truth teller" and it said that he did not really want closeness and physical intimacy with a woman he felt was destroying him.

There are other examples, some so transparent that they are amusing. For example, an obviously hostile woman who was always putting down men, recently asked me if I could confirm her experience that "just about all men today have impotency problems." Clearly, she was not aware of the impact her hostility toward men had on her lovers. She apparently believed that erections automatically appear under all conditions. Her underlying assumption was that men have no emotional reactions when it comes to sex, and that a "normal" man will automatically have an erection when there is a naked, willing woman.

Men are not impotent today. They only are impotent with *some* women under *some* conditions and their non-responsive reactions reflect important truths that they must learn to trust and understand.

In all of these examples, and in a myriad of others, the man was ready to blame himself totally or to search for "deep" and hidden meanings in his past. Certain kinds of contemporary conditioning techniques and "helpful" and "supportive" advice such as "You know you don't have to get an erection each and every time. Just lay back and let it happen," would have done these men great disservice. Their basic distrust of the wisdom of their body responses would only have been reinforced.

There are fewer sights more sad than a man who was once so joyously potent and has since become "impotent" acting desperately grateful for the return of his erection, no matter what the price. He is suddenly willing to have his erection on any terms just to recoup his "self-respect," even if he has to manipulate, twist, and distort his sensibilities totally to accomplish this. I don't believe that an erection, no matter how achieved, is a good thing simply because it reduces a man's anxiety for the moment. I feel that this attitude robs him of the necessity of owning up to his real feelings about his partner or the relationship in which he's involved. The man who gets his erections by cheating on himself through fantasizing sex with other women, arousing himself with pornography, or using various and sundry mechanical devices is demonstrating disrespect for himself and rejection of his real emotions.

I feel strongly that a man only have sex under conditions of genuine total spontaneous excitement and full arousal. With anything short of that reaction he may be setting the groundwork for impotence. The penis is not a piece of plumbing that functions capriciously. It is an expression of the total self. In these days of over-intellectualization it is perhaps the only remaining sensitive and revealing barometer of the male's true sexual feelings. A man's conscious brain is awash with guilt-making messages and rationalizations when he is not able to "perform." He accuses himself in a self-deprecating manner with phrases like, "I'm hostile and non-giving," "I'm sexually inadequate," "I'm afraid of closeness," "I'm not good enough for her and am incapable of satisfying her," "I'm not a man," or "Maybe I love her too much and can only perform when I'm rejected." All these self-accusations disguise the immediate reality of his feelings and/or his partner's. By ignoring, rationalizing away, or trying to disguise his lack of genuine sexual response, the man is giving up a large and critical part of himself and demonstrating self-hate. By taking responsibility for his feelings and encouraging his partner to do likewise he can begin to overcome the fantasy of impotence as exclusively a male "problem."

The Monogamy Question

One of the most critical problems the contemporary male has in expressing his authentic sexual response is that, due to a negative image of himself as a promiscuous, lustful animal (graphically expressed in the common saying "an erect penis has no conscience"), he has tried to conform to standards of monogamous sexual involvement that are alien to his early conditioning. This conditioning creates the foundation for guilt and performance anxiety. In our culture, the young man is conditioned to *challenge and conquer* in the sexual arena. He is reinforced heavily by his teenage peers for his ability to "make" as many girls as he can. Whether this is "healthy" or not, it is nevertheless his emotional and social heritage, one which he struggles against, valiantly tries to overcome, and often hates himself for. Traditionally, most females, on the other hand, have been conditioned to view sex as a part of total love relationship that leads to permanency and marriage.

In one sense, therefore, sex in marriage conflicts with the male's powerful early conditioning. However, he learns that his conditioning, his style, and his needs are "shallow" or "bad" and that her motives are somehow correct—and purer. When he feels inclined to stray or "cheat," he ultimately and invariably is bombarded with guilt and self-hating messages.

Expressed in another way, the man and woman in a perma-

nent, exclusive relationship may be having sex at cross purposes. For him, traditionally, sex has meant challenge and
conquest and a variety of women. This is missing in marriage.
For her, sex meant belonging, intimacy, and security. Because
men invariably try to accommodate female needs rather than
fulfill their own, whether "right" or "wrong," "good" or
"bad," they will live, as in Thoreau's description, ". . . lives
of quiet desperation."[4] Only when the marriage finally ends,
when and if it does, is the male able to fully feel and admit the
intense sexual frustration he had been experiencing throughout the marital relationship.

Another aspect of long-range male-female relationships that
tends to undermine satisfaction within a monogamous sexual
relationship is hidden aggression. That is, the romantic orientation and conditioning to suppress and repress direct and
open assertion of needs and the free expression of anger inevitably results in sex being used as a weapon. The relationship,
by being laden with repressed negative feelings, becomes increasingly more distant and cold. The "nice" male lover,
therefore, becomes less passionate, spontaneous, and close to
his wife or partner.

The phenomenon of mother transference is another powerful barrier to sexual satisfaction within the marital relationship. Our culture has become largely matriarchal. In most
cases, father has become a secondary part of the family structure. Often he is working at one of two jobs or is glued to the
television set. Or, he is preoccupied and worried and lacks
energy when he is at home. If the family has been broken up
by divorce, chances are that mother has custody.

Consequently, the boy develops deep dependencies and iden-
tifications with mother. His feelings toward her must inevitably be in conflict. While she loves and nurtures him she also
sets his limits and restricts him. And though she is the most
important person in his life, sexual feelings toward her are
taboo. When the male marries and his wife begins to assume
many of the fuctions of a mothering figure—feeding him, taking care of his clothing, caring for the house and the children—he inevitably develops some mother transferences to
her and this has to dampen erotic aspects of the relationship.

While there may be many satisfying aspects to a marital
relationship for many men, sex may just not be one of them.
The male is therefore in a crisis in marriage. As a liberated

human being who is entitled to the deep fulfillment of his needs just as a woman is to hers, he will have to acknowledge and come to terms with his own unique sexual rhythm and desires or pay the price of having sundry psychosomatic and psychological symptoms.

Polygamy is the norm in twice as many cultures as monogamy.[5] The revitalizing impact of a new sex partner is widely accepted. Many so-called impotent, passive, or disinterested men find themselves extremely potent with a new partner. Research has indicated that married people tend to have frequent intercourse with their mates only at the beginning of the sexual relationship. The frequency greatly diminishes as time passes. Even Kinsey's now-out-dated study indicated that approximately three-fourths of the married men interviewed expressed desires for extra-marital affairs and 50 per cent acknowledged having indulged in them.[6] (The invigorating effect of new sex partners was the subject of a humorous anecdote involving Calvin Coolidge. The story goes that the late President Coolidge was reportedly observing some barnyard activity with his First Lady when she commented on the impressive sexual powers of the males. In responding to the truth of her observation, the President pointed out that the males never stayed with the same partner.)[7]

The word "cheating" in marriage is a particularly unfortunate one. It has extremely negative connotations, like the word "stealing." A man humiliates himself when he "cheats"—when he sneaks around rather than openly having an affair. The whole process of lying and covering up tracks is degrading. It only serves to validate his hostile self-image of being a "bad boy" or a promiscuous, lusting beast.

The married man who desires other women, therefore, may have to learn to emancipate himself by acting out his sexual desires more openly and guiltlessly and discussing his needs and feelings honestly with his wife. He needs to come to look at his sexual appetite as a part of his unique make-up and openly own up to being who he is. Nor need this be an exercise in male chauvinism. That is, he also needs to learn to accept his wife's unique sexual rhythm, whatever that may be. A recent study conducted in a suburban town indicated that, given the appropriate opportunity, over two-thirds of the men and 56 per cent of the women had a high potential for extra-marital sexual intercourse.[8]

A psychoanalyst and the author of a recent book on male survival said of men: "By the time he reaches his forties, this statistic [sexual intercourse] is reduced to 1.5 weekly coital connections. He spends more time shaving than he does copulating."⁹ Surely, the male is cheating himself of a vital joy and is entitled to reclaim his full share of the primal pleasures of sex.

The man in our culture lives under much stress that is difficult or impossible to avoid or control. His sex life, however, can be in his control. While the monogamy question is admittedly complex and emotionally loaded, the male doesn't have to conform to a model of sexual behavior that is antithetic to his own needs. For too many married men, sex in marriage becomes just another job, a duty or responsibility he feels it is his obligation to fulfill. And to add insult to injury he sees it as a test of his ability to perform. It doesn't have to be that way if he is willing to risk owning up to his identity. Liberating himself sexually means that he will reclaim his right to function sexually in a way that is fulfilling and genuine.

Fusion Sex

Recently I have been exploring the possibility of different kinds of intensities of male orgasms and sexual experiences. I brought the issue up at a marathon psychotherapy session two years ago and discovered that not all but a number of men had experienced what I have come to term "fusion sex."

The experience of fusion sex is one of an intense, totally un-self-conscious sexual coming together during which the male is not focusing on or aware of having sex per se but is simply a part of a wholly spontaneous, ecstatic union or fusion with the female, one that often brings him to tears of joy.

In fusion sex there is the phenomenon of a seemingly endless potency, lasting sometimes for an entire weekend or several days during which time he remains in bed making love continually. Men who have reported fusion sex to me describe the phenomenon of ejaculating and then almost immediately becoming erect again. They may have as many as twelve to fifteen orgasms during a weekend's experience of fusion sex. Indeed, the cup overfloweth.

The common ingredients to fusion sex that men who have experienced it describe are:

1) The man either recently has left a long-standing though frustrating sexual relationship or has been looking for a truly satisfying one without success for a long time. In a word, he is ripe.

2) The fusion sex relationship is not predicated on a future potential. Neither party has long-range designs on the other. The woman may be married and intending to return to her husband or living in another part of the country or world and planning to go back shortly. In other words, there are serious obstacles to permanency, the future is highly uncertain, and therefore the relationship is totally *now*.

3) The male is flooded with and able to experience and express long-repressed feelings that never or very rarely emerge. That is, during fusion sex he is able to cry in sadness, to experience his loneliness, to cling, to be passive, to enjoy feeling beautiful and to be totally transparent about his fantasies, his feelings, his past, and his future aspirations. In short, he is temporarily whole, reunited with long lost parts of himself.

4) The male senses a real challenge. He has found his "magic lady" who is not free or readily available and he is totally expressive in his pursuit and desire for her.

The most important aspects of this apparently exquisite relationship-experience are that it is totally in the present. There are no strings attached and no future plans. The male feels sufficiently safe and accepted. He can become emotionally defenseless and allow a total flow of blocked and typically controlled feelings to emerge. In most cases that I have heard of, such relationships did not gain permanence. They never had to meet the long range test of "reality."

I have also heard of a few instances of fusion sex occurring for a man who has been in a relationship with a woman for many years. Usually it seems to happen for him after a personal growth crisis which has allowed him to achieve new levels of awareness. In these periods he is able to experience new levels of trust leading to greater self-expression which then allows him to surrender himself more completely to the sexual moment and therefore to experience the ecstasy of fusion sex.

The experience of fusion sex is certainly deserving of further exploration. It may very well have been experienced by men under conditions quite dissimilar to the ones outlined here, and I don't want to imply that the dimensions I've discussed are the only ones. However, hearing descriptions of this experience leads me to believe that most men have not experienced nearly the ecstatic potential of their sexuality. While I am not suggesting that the male set fusion sex as a constant standard of expectation, descriptions of the experience of fusion sex certainly do contain important implications for the untapped sexual potential of the male.

Symbol Sex or The Male As Sex Object

One major accusation most frequently hurled at men is that they treat women like faceless sex objects. Men, however, are the recipients of a different and equally virulent form of this style of relating which I term "symbol sex." Whereas a man may indeed have a tendency to respond to a woman on the basis of her physical appearance, the woman's attraction to a man is often based on his status, income, and power. One well-known actress, famous for marrying millionaires and dating major political figures and famous performers, verbalized it aptly and honestly: "Men I like have two things in common—they are smart and they have power."[10] Men who react with guilt to the accusation that they are treating a woman like a sex object seem to take this woman's attitude for granted, without any awareness of its implications. It confirms the destructive self-concept that if they have no money or a low-status job they don't deserve the "high class" women.

A depressed young man of twenty-four came to me for therapy. He viewed himself as a professional failure and as someone who was undesirable to women. Women consistently rejected his sexual advances even though he was attractive physically.

I suggested that he participate in a marathon encounter growth group, which he did. In the group he also did not draw much female attention. Subsequently, however, he became fascinated with these group experiences and enrolled in a training course to become a para-professional facilitator. During the very first group session in which the leader announced that this young man was his assistant, in training to be a leader, female response to him changed dramatically. Before the twenty-four-hour group experience was over two of the most attractive women present had openly indicated their sexual interest in him. Bathed in the aura of power he had suddenly become sexually transformed.

The groupie phenomenon in the world of rock 'n' roll is an extreme form of symbol sex. Groupies are females, from early teenagers to considerably older women, who make themselves sexually available to famous rock singers and on occasion even whole groups. In fact, sometimes all it takes to go to bed with a groupie is to be a star's friend or an employee who is able to help facilitate contact with the star. A California free-lance writer recalled one such experience when he was touring with the singing group, the Rolling Stones. A girl walked through his door and asked him if he was a friend of the Stones. When he replied that he was, she took off her clothes and lay down on the bed.[11]

While the groupie phenomenon may represent an extreme, like a man who can only love a girl with big breasts, it still reflects a very real and hazardous fact of male experience. For example, whether an older man who pursues a younger woman is a "dirty old man," or "hip and interesting," often boils down to the issue of his money and his position. One of the very first questions single women ask each other when discussing their dates is "What does he do?" A doctor is considered a good catch; a high school graduate blue collar worker is not, even if the latter may have much more to give emotionally and sexually than the former.

Symbol sex presents a special hazard to a man in that it increases his sense of alienation and isolation. Deep inside himself he knows that his attractiveness to a woman is closely linked to his continuing ability to succeed in the outside world. He knows that if he loses status, power, or money he stands to lose sexual attractiveness and love as well.

The male thus finds himself in an impossible bind. If he continues to pursue success vigorously he has less capacity for involvement in his love relationship. If he does not pursue success vigorously, he becomes less desirable.

Masters and Johnson, while discussing the female surrogates whom they hired to work with their sexually dysfunctional males, were quoted as saying, "You could call it coincidence if you like, but we never had a surrogate become emotionally involved with a man who didn't have money."[12]

Prostitution As Male Humiliation

Feminists have expressed the idea that prostitution is an exercise in male chauvinism, one that results in the degradation of the female wherein she is simultaneously being exploited by her customers, her pimp, and the police.

While there is merit to this argument, there is still hardly a more humiliating, self-annihilating and less satisfying experience for a man than a visit to a prostitute, an experience that thoroughly reinforces the hateful self-image of himself as a despicable animal.

To be sure, not all prostitutes are the same. Some are more sensitive, supportive, and emotionally atuned than others. However, even under the best of conditions a man tends to leave this experience with his worst conscious thoughts about himself as a person confirmed.

A friend of mine was describing his first sexual experience, which happened to have been with a prostitute. He was fifteen-years-old and living in a time when sex with a girl friend was still not common. The prostitute he went to was not a high-class call girl, nor was she a streetwalker. Appointments were made by telephone and the customer rang the apartment buzzer three times as a signal to let him in.

I came into her apartment on West End Avenue in New York City. There was one older dude sitting in the kitchen and another guy waiting in the hallway. She was in the bedroom screwing but came to the door. She told me to wait in the kitchen with the older dude. We sat there waiting our turns and trying to avoid looking at each other—obviously we both felt ashamed to be there.

Twenty minutes later she called me in. She asked me for my ten dollars first. After I got undressed she washed me like a baby with soap and water and then put a rubber on me and believe it or not started to blow me with the damn thing on. I couldn't feel a thing. About two minutes later, at the most, she asked me if I was "ready" yet because she couldn't spend all day with me. Before I could answer, she got on her back, spread her legs and put some saliva in her vagina to lubricate herself. As soon as I was inside she started going "ooh" and "aah" trying to convince me, I guess, that I was really turning her on. Meanwhile, she wouldn't even let me kiss her and she wouldn't let me put my fingers into her. She said that she was too sore. In the middle of her "oohing" and "aahing" the telephone rang. She answered it while I was still inside of her and casually made another appointment for that day—she even gave the guy instructions on how many times to ring the bell.

When she got done with her phone call she asked me impatiently if I was "finished" yet. When I said "no" she got pissed off. She told me that I better hurry up. This was only about nine minutes and one phone call after I had come into the room. Finally she got me to come by removing the rubber and jerking me off. Then she hustled me out of the room and made me put my clothes on in the hall.

Listen to Laurie, a twenty-three-year-old prostitute, who expresses the contemptuous attitude that many men will receive during a visit to a prostitute. Her techniques were described by a writer who had interviewed her:

She insists that she be allowed to wash a man whom she is about to sleep with—"With me it's none of this 'You go into the bathroom . . . and wash yourself' stuff, 'cause they don't do it. They'll sprinkle a little water and say they're clean," she says contemptuously, "but they're not." It's hot water and soap with Laurie and she maintains that it is indeed necessary. . . .

Following her clinical ministrations, she magically clicks on the role of a John's 'long lost lover.' That's part of being a hooker: "You have to act like you're in love with them and tell them how good it is . . . I have no sensation or feeling, no nothing . . . Most of them make me sick, though," she says.[13]

The manner in which Laurie perceives her customers is indeed humiliating to the male.

Not surprisingly, a good proportion of the customers of prostitutes are not single men with no women but married men. The married men who frequent prostitutes are all too often men who are trying to live up to the demands of a "meaningful relationship" and who have become super self-conscious in their inhibited sensitivity, "gentleness," and restrained behavior with their wives. They are starved for a moment of spontaneous, nonobligating, aggressively free sexual abandon. They go off and buy it, but the price is further damage to their already negative male self-image.

The answers to this problem are, of course, fairly complex and difficult to sort out. Many men have been so negatively conditioned and inhibited that they no longer seem to be able to be spontaneously sexual in an intimate relationship. This harks back to early memories of being called "horny" or feeling like an animal because they aggressively lusted after a "nice" girl. Surely, the changes in the male psyche will require a revolution in the evaluation of his sexual patterns and desires.

Male Homosexuality

Most "straight" males are terrified of the experience of homosexuality, no matter how liberated they may be in their thinking. Reports on heterosexual group-sex experiences invariably indicate that the men studiously avoid sexual contact with each other, preferring instead to watch the women have sex between themselves. Trio sex almost always means two women and one man. When two men and one woman make up the group the men usually both play with the woman and then take turns having sex with her, all the while avoiding contact with each other.

It is my observation, shared by many of my colleagues, that women seem to be far less threatened by homosexual contact. In fact, in some of the more sophisticated quarters bisexuality has become an "in" thing for women. One recent article described this burgeoning phenomenon. It suggested that in some circles it is even socially undesirable for a woman to be afraid to try sex with another woman.[14]

Males however continue to be frozen in their response to each other. This is understandable. The culture has a much more hostile and punitive attitude toward male homosexuals. A recent study pointed out that the greatest proportion of legal harassment and over 90 per cent of the arrests on charge of homosexuality involve male homosexuals. Perhaps the male homosexual is more visible than the female. However, another critical factor is that our culture is still mired in very negative and distorted perceptions regarding him. One twenty-three year-old male homosexual, a computer operator, expressed it to me this way: "There are a lot of men who really get uptight around me. They think, 'Oh my God, he's sick. He needs a doctor,' or 'Put him away somewhere,' or 'He lurks in the bushes molesting little kids.' "

Every male brought up in a traditional home develops an intense early identification with his mother and therefore carries within him a strong feminine imprint. The opposite is not true of the female whose attachment to and therefore identification with her father is usually not nearly as intense as the male's to his mother. Therefore, it would seem that men would be considerably more likely to act out homosexually than women. In fact, the whole phenomenon of macho can be interpreted as a strong male reaction against the feminine component within himself because of his intense fear of it.

The dilemma was well stated in *Gay Mystique*. In it Peter Fisher wrote:

> The masculine role is defensive. Men are to be hollow fortresses, safe from attack or loss of status from without, safe from inappropriate emotions and uncertainty from within. American men are not encouraged to know other men. We think of women as intuitive, possibly because they are permitted to stay in touch with their deeper feelings to a much greater extent than men.[15]

While I am not advocating casual experimentation with homosexuality for males, being highly aware of the intense anxieties and repression that block these impulses, it is extremely critical for the sake of male survival that every man integrate into consciousness the powerful feminine aspects that exist within himself. The immense masculine defenses against homosexual impulses are life-draining, creating a fear of passivity that may drive the male into endless, exhausting rounds of activity in order to defend himself against these impulses. This is undoubtedly a factor in the shorter life-span of the male. He is more resistant to sleeping, lying in bed when he doesn't feel well, allowing someone else to take care of him, or just doing nothing.

The female component also demands integration into the male psyche because unconscious homosexual panic may create many serious emotional symptoms that occasionally even result in suicide. The real underlying homosexual impulses

and fears in the man rarely surface openly to his consciousness. Rather, the typical pattern is one in which a man who is
abandoned by a female lover or becomes impotent is suddenly
flooded with intense anxiety and despair. One important result
of this may be the threatened surfacing of unconscious homosexual impulses. To allay the anxieties he turns to drinking
heavily or indulging in reckless, self-destructive macho-style
behavior such as driving at high speeds or frantically trying
to pick up women.

Only with the integration of his feminine, passive side will
the male be able to liberate himself sexually, allowing himself
to experience the totality of his feelings and freeing himself
from concerns about performance and dominance. The macho
male is an incomplete, dull heterosexual partner because he
clings so heavily to his stereotypical ways of responding.

Guidelines For The Sexual Liberation
Of The Male

1. Do not participate in sex unless you are fully aroused.
   Never fake involvement or perform half-heartedly to be
   "nice." This may be the beginning of so-called impotence
   and the end of joyful, lustful, total sexuality.
2. Learn to say "no" if you have no desire. You are not a sex
   machine and it is no reflection on your adequacy as a
   male. Therefore, don't apologize, lie, or make excuses instead of saying, "No, I don't feel like it."
3. Forget all the old imperatives regarding male obligations to
   satisfy the female. Do not preoccupy yourself with her orgasms or try to divine her needs. Instead, focus on your
   own responses and pleasure.
4. Respect, cherish, listen, and learn from your body's responses. If you get no erection do not become anxious. Ask
   yourself what your body is trying to tell you that you are
   not consciously telling yourself. Most important, respect
   the wisdom of your penis. Your goal is not to be potent,
   but rather to be true to your responses and to learn from
   and take full responsibility for the truth of your feelings.
5. Do not preoccupy yourself with techniques. If you do, ask

yourself if you are not really experiencing a lack of passion or its demise. The finest "technique" is a fully aroused body. Do not confuse techniques for the essence of the sexual experience.

6. Get in touch with your feminine side. Allow yourself to be sexually passive as well as active. Let her make love to you and take some of the lead. Lie back and enjoy it.

7. Finally, remember that potentially there are two free, responsible, assertive people in bed. Do not degrade her or yourself by treating her like a fragile flower. Assert your needs and share your feelings and trust that she will do likewise.

4. Feelings:
The Real Male Terror

As they worked through months of interview sessions together . . . Buzz (Aldrin) relived many painful aspects of his life: The achievement-oriented education as a West Point cadet, the single-mindedness of the Air Force hierarchy, the hypocrisy of the NASA astronaut publicity, the illusions of heroism, the cracks in his family life, and finally, his emotional breakdown.[1]

The male hero image in our culture is reflected in the men who constitute our fantasy identification figures. Most of them share certain specific characteristics: emotional mutedness or "cool," an extremely independent style, self-containment, or lack of transparency or apparent emotional vulnerability, and in general, a very narrow band of outward expressiveness.

A group of eighty college men were asked by researchers to indicate their preferred heroes. As reported, they invariably preferred stories of males who were solitary, strong, independent, and in the process of actively striving to overcome obstacles. The heroes rarely gave signs of seeking out close relationships with people, although they did occasionally bestow on them a kind of impersonal attention, one which further served to demonstrate their own greater adequacy.[2]

Today, despite often-heard verbalizations to the contrary and an emphasis on feelings which has emerged from the world of encounter and growth groups, there is still great discomfort and embarrassment when a man overtly and spontaneously expresses his emotions, breaks down in tears, rages in open anger or hate, trembles and shakes in fear, or even laughs too boisterously. Occasionally, when male political leaders show spontaneous emotion their images become tarnished and they lose points, as when Senator Muskie openly lost his temper during the 1972 campaign, vice-presidential candidate Tom Eagleton was revealed to have experienced depressions, President Johnson pulled on the ears of his dog or showed the world his post-operative scar, or Kissinger lost his cool at a press conference.

The alleged social encouragement for men to express feelings more freely is still largely in the abstract. Even when men get together in their own "liberation groups" they often become rather quickly mired in intellectualizations and platitudes, and the interactions are seldom spontaneous and genuine on a feeling level.

The contemporary preoccupation with feelings and the stress on their expression is a reflection of how repressed, unavailable, and rare a genuine feeling is. Real feelings are apparently so hard to come by that our culture is handsomely supporting a whole new profession of feeling facilitators. These are persons who are paid for granting permission and providing a setting for the expression and exploration of feelings.

Unfortunately, however, research suggests that the carryover from group to the outside world is too often minimal. Clearly, the male is still in a cultural climate that has little authentic tolerance for his emotional expressiveness. Picture, if you will, the possible reactions to a man at work who cries at his desk over the loss of a sale. Or picture the response to a man who caresses fellow male employees, who expresses rage toward an employer, who openly announces that he wishes to be passive and allow others to carry the ball for him, or confesses to and indulges his feelings of fear over a challenging job responsibility. Even in his personal life, among friends or with his wife, the tolerance for his "letting go" and freely expressing feelings is very limited and must be preceded with a justification, i.e., "I think I'm entitled to get angry," and followed by an apology.

The autonomous male, the independent strong achiever who can be counted on to be always in control is still essentially the preferred male image. Success in the working world is predicated on the repression of self and the display of a controlled, deliberate, calculated, manipulative responsiveness. To become a leader requires that one be totally goal-oriented, undistracted by personal factors, and able to tune out extraneous "noise," human or otherwise, which is unrelated to the end goal and which might impede forward motion. The man who "feels" becomes inefficient and ineffective because he gets emotionally involved and this inevitably slows him down and distracts him. His more dehumanized competitor will then surely pass him by.

The behavior of many contemporary men is in some ways analogous to the behavior patterns of autistic children. The autistic child's responses are an extreme form of resistance to human contact, with a concomitant extreme fascination and fixation on inanimate objects. Touching another person, expressing feelings, and relating to others are traumatic and largely avoided. Contemporary man is encapsulated in the world of his automobile, which may get more genuine concern and involvement than any human being in his life. Or, he is staring at his television, transistor radio plugged into his ear, stereo piping through earphones, a newspaper or magazine hiding his face, stimulated by liquor, cigarettes, and pills, aroused by pornography, eating frozen or pre-packaged foods, hitting golf balls at the driving range, and negotiating his life in two-minute spurts over the telephone. He can truly and comfortably keep himself stimulated with only the barest human contact for days or weeks on end. In fact, human contact may even be experienced as an irritating intrusion; interference with his television watching or while he's working on his automobile is sure to arouse his wrath. He may even have sex, after the first few weeks of a relationship, lying prone in front of the television, timing his orgasm to occur during the commercials so that no time is lost from his involvement with the program.

One of our key culture heroes is the laboratory scientist, a man who can "tune out" the world and literally spend days on end working in his laboratory with only his computer, his reactor, his microscope, or his chemicals for companionship. The feeling male with ongoing interpersonal needs would find such work unbearable.

The male has become anesthetized and robotized because he has been heavily socialized to repress and deny almost the total range of his emotions and human needs in order that he can perform in the acceptable "masculine" way. Feelings become unknown, unpredictable quantities, expression of which threaten him and make him feel vulnerable. By the time he is a mature adult he also has undoubtedly surrounded himself with a family environment that has a heavy stake in his continuing non-feeling and in subtle ways reinforces his functioning as a well-oiled machine. Should inner feelings come pouring through, particularly on a continuing basis, in the form of powerful emotional needs, fears, and conflicts, he would be encouraged to get professional help to patch him up and help him regain control.

Some women who I hear complaining and wishing that their men would express more feelings remind me of the wives of alcoholics who protest how much they want their husbands to stop drinking, or the wives of successful men who say they wish their success-driven husbands would slow down, work less, and relate more. Should their wishes ever come true they often unconsciously obstruct the change in some passive or indirect way and push their husbands back into their old patterns.

One such success-driven male decided to cut down on his work and stay home more. After a few days of his euphoria over this newly found free time, he was driven back to hard work again by his absence of genuine interests, his impatience with the children, his wife's compulsive housework routines, the boredom of his marriage, which he didn't fully recognize while he was working, and the total absence of sensuality with his wife which, previously, he had always been conveniently able to blame on fatigue from overwork. His wife, despite her protestations, was happier than he was that he was going back to work. Without him conquering and bringing home the spoils there was really nothing of meaning in the relationship.

What emotions, impulses, and needs is the male blocking? The answer, I believe, seems to be *more or less all of them.* Almost from infancy on he is taught to control the expression of feelings and needs that interfere with the masculine style of goal-directed, task-oriented, self-assertive behavior. That is, in the emotional area his socialization experience was "Thou shalt not." Systematically, in direct or subtle ways, feelings and impulses were constantly being suppressed.

Dependency

A boy who clings to his parents is an embarrassment. He is encouraged in countless ways from early boyhood on to cut the apron strings. The little girl however, who bashfully hides and holds onto her mother or father, is seen as cute or adorable.

Dependency in the male is equated with weakness, so much so that even normal amounts are often suppressed. There is little that makes a father prouder than to see his five or six-year-old son acting like a "little man."

The male child's dependency needs are equally as verboten when directed at mother or at father. If his mother tolerates or encourages them, she stands to be accused of emasculating him. Father, ever mindful of the competitive struggles of his everyday life, overreacts and sees his son's dependency as dangerous. His survival philosophy of "never count on anybody but yourself" makes the expression of dependency the equivalent of "loser" and "victim." "That's my boy!" is never said in reference to dependent behavior, but only in response to signs of self-sufficiency and vigorous independence.

From early childhood on the boy learns that masculinity means not depending on anybody. His needs are bottled up and disowned. He reacts violently to those who lean on others and calls them "parasites." When he himself is forced into a position of having to depend on someone else he becomes anxious and distrustful, certain that he will be let down. Dependency, in the typical male mind, spells disaster.

Passivity

Laying back and doing nothing is extremely threatening to the male who has learned to equate masculinity with activity, striving, competing, and overcoming obstacles. Passivity, in his perception, is equivalent to feminity. He expects to be Tom Sawyer walking the picket fence while Becky watches and admires him from the sidelines.

From early boyhood on, he is pressed to produce, to be adventurous, to stay in motion, and to have unlimited energy. If he sits passively in the corner reading, his parents worry and wonder about him. Most boys have a voice inside of themselves, driving them on and admonishing them to, "Get off your tail and *do* something!"

As an adult, with his need to be passive now totally repressed, he becomes unhappy and anxious if he has to sit around and "do nothing." Time that is not channeled into goal-directed behavior or some kind of "productive" work is considered wasted. He can only be passive on occasion, when he is rewarding himself for a long stretch of hard work and he can tell himself that he "earned it."

The resistance against passivity and the tendency toward incessant activity becomes an end in itself, one that makes every accomplishment unsatisfying and hollow because the male is unable to lie back and enjoy his fruits. Where he may have originally rationalized his constant activity as assuring him a secure future, when that future comes he is unable to enjoy it because he is too threatened by passivity. He therefore creates the fantasy that he is doing it for his wife and children. This justifies further activity.

A close friend related how a woman he had recently met had actively courted him. She telephoned and told him how attractive she found him to be. She told him directly that she wanted to have him for dinner and then to make love to him. He was charmed and excited and accepted the invitation.

When he arrived she poured him champagne, brought him food, and played romantic music on the stereo. But when it came to having sex she had one request. She wanted to do it her way and at her pace. She would tell him what she wanted him to do, how she wanted it done, and when. However, being passive in this way, he found himself feeling increasingly uptight and uncomfortable. Even though he was fulfilling a long-held fantasy of being actively seduced by a woman he admitted later that he found the experience "painfully unbearable."

The inability to tolerate passivity also destroys the natural alternating life rhythm of activity followed by passivity. This is undoubtedly one major cause of many men being burnt out or being afflicted by chronic diseases at an early age. The repression of the passive dimension prevents the regularly needed time for rest and recovery.

Asking for Help

The male resistance to asking for help ties in closely with both his resistance to dependency and his resistance to passivity. As a boy he learns that a major indicator of "manliness" is to be able to say, "I can do it by myself. I don't need anybody's help." "God helps those who help themselves," is a singularly male attitude. Having to ask for help makes him feel uncomfortable, anxious, and vulnerable.

As a boy he may struggle for hours over a problem or task because he is too embarrassed to ask for help. As an adult he may drive around lost for a half-hour, hoping to stumble on the right direction rather than to stop and ask for help. He hides his business and other worldly problems because he's convinced that no one can help him anyway. Others might, he thinks, even use his helplessness *against* him.

In the less tangible areas of interpersonal and emotional problems he is loathe to turn to a friend or even a professional and say, "Please help me. I can't carry on anymore." Instead, he suffers and struggles in silence and when he finally breaks down or, in extreme cases, commits suicide, often even his intimates are surprised. They weren't aware anything was wrong.

If he finally goes to a psychotherapist he tries to transform it into a task-oriented experience rather than a relationship experience. He wants to be taught as efficiently and quickly as possible "How to. . . ," and thereby get the process over with as efficiently as possible.

His resistance against asking for help tends to devastate his relationships with intimates, spouse, friends, and children. If they love him, he believes, they will know what he needs. They will magically "divine" him without his having to ask for help. He quietly resents it when they don't. He broods in secret silence and turns himself off from them even more. "No one really cares. They just want to use me," he says to himself. This steels him even more, reassuring him that he is right in his perception that no one is going to help him.

Fear

Words like "chicken-shit," "scaredy cat," "coward," "gutless," "no balls," and "sissy" ring in the male's ear a lifetime and often drive him into senseless, self-destructive, even crazy behaviors and risk-taking in order to prove to himself and others, over and over again, that he is a man and that he isn't afraid.

As a young boy he was praised for having "guts" if he fought a boy considerably bigger than himself. Nothing could fill him with pride more than to hear it said of himself, "Nothing scares him," or "He's not afraid of anything." The highest compliment would be to call him "fearless."

The inner pressure to deny fear—the fear of acknowledging fear—leads to many kinds of self-destructive activities. A challenging look or a word wrongly uttered will justify a fight with a stranger. Many of the unnecessary things a man does such as climbing a dangerous mountain, speeding on a motorcycle, taking on an onerous job, may be done to fight the feeling of fear. But he dare not give in to his fears or he couldn't live with his self-accusations. His victories therefore are often hollow because they were motivated by the negative impulse to deny the feeling of fear in himself. That need is insatiable and he will continue to push himself to prove again and again that he is fearless.

I often have had to use all of my own rational controls to prevent myself from jumping out of my automobile in traffic to meet the challenge of someone who has made an obscene gesture to me. Then I have to reassure myself that I'm not a coward for having done so, even though to do so would have been totally self-destructive and stupid.

The chivalrous attitude of one male fighting another male who has insulted a woman companion is another variation on this self-destructive theme. Hopefully, the increasing liberation of the female will convince the male that she is not a fragile, helpless being who is destroyed by a remark and that she is fully capable of responding on her own behalf if she so chooses.

Sadness and Tears

The echoes of "Big boys don't cry," and "Crybaby!" resonate deep within the male psyche and block the flow of tears and the full experience of sadness. One twenty-three-year-old patient of mine described his early experience as follows, "When I was twelve years old my father mocked me for crying one time. I consciously made a decision right then and there that I would never cry again. And I kept it too, for years. When I finally realized crying is good, and that men need to cry too, I couldn't do it any more. Since then I've been trying to learn to cry again, and it's been very difficult. The same thing goes for other feelings. It's very hard for me to let myself experience them most of the time."

There is something about a male in tears, whether as a boy or as a man that offends, causes others to turn away and to want to "do something" to stop it as soon as possible. Tears from a woman bring out a protective feeling. From a male, tears create discomfort at best and occasionally even mild disgust at his inability to "control himself." Manliness is still equated with poise and composure in the face of tragedy. A man who is often in tears seems to everyone, including himself, to be falling apart, or to be having a "nervous breakdown." It is only through a conscious act of will that the liberated person can sit comfortably with a man and let him cry himself out, particularly if he does so on a fairly frequent basis. The first time may be all right. But the third or fourth time is neurotic, infantile, or at least annoying and unpleasant.

Aggression

Supposedly, aggression is one area of expression expected and approved of in the male. In reality in turns out to be just another taboo area.

From early boyhood on everyone expects the male to be aggressive. The expression of it is however, expected to be nonpersonal, directed against strangers, competitors, enemies, and other outside targets. At home or in school the boy's aggression is severely curtailed. He is not allowed to talk back, to lose his temper, to be boisterous, to insult, to confront, or to fight.

In interaction with their intimates the most vicious killers and ruthless businessmen have often been described as gentle, kind, sweet individuals who wouldn't hurt a fly.

In a sense, the male is forced into a Jekyll and Hyde type of behavior. He shows his aggressive face only to those who are not close to him. This creates a dangerous situation. Assuming that a certain amount of aggression is inherent in each man, the ethics of aggression force him to find non-personal outlets or targets. He behaves irrationally, viciously, and cruelly as he displaces his aggression away from the real source onto "suitable" targets.

Anger Toward Women

Males learn very early in life that psychologically they will lose any confrontation with a female, because win or lose they will be labeled "bullies." As a young boy he is castigated for fighting with his sister. He is taught that the female is fragile and that he is to be her protector, never her opponent or competitor. Her tendency to cry rather than to assert herself directly often results in a male reaction of guilt.

As an adult, the inability to get angry at a female without "righteous" cause such as her "cheating" on him, insulting his masculinity, or not feeding him on time, prevents him from relating to her on an equal basis. The traditional male unconsciously and defensively reacts against this anger, and the emotion becomes transformed into a super-macho overprotection of her, in which he perceives her as much more fragile, childlike, and helpless than she is in reality. That defense will cause him to rush to do battle on her behalf for totally irrational and self-destructive reasons.

Second, the defense against anger will spell the death of spontaneous sexuality. In his need to be super-gentle and super-sensitive, to reassure her and himself that he harbors no aggressive feelings toward her, he paralyzes himself and also encourages her to role-play the gentle madonna in order to collude with his fantasy.

Third, the defense against the expression of anger will make him very guilt-prone in relationship to her. He will be easily manipulated by tears or acts of helplessness that produce in him self-accusations of "sadist" whenever he is vigorously assertive or loses his temper toward her.

Finally, the aggression and anger toward her that he has denied and defended himself against will emerge in countless indirect and hidden ways in the form of detachment and withdrawal, psychosomatic complaints, and sundry other passive forms of aggression.

The feminist movement has focused attention on this situation. The liberated woman has broken her traditional pattern and become overtly assertive and aggressive in relation to the male. He however, is still frozen in fear of his own anger toward her and consequently has reponded to her accusations and villifications primarily with guilt and pitiful intellectualized attempts to reform himself to please her. At the same time the rage he is not expressing directly is emerging as a steadily decreasing capacity and willingness to relate in an intimate one-to-one, enduring way. He is now being told that he is afraid of the woman. What he is *really* afraid of are his own impulses of anger and rage toward her over being increasingly abandoned, frustrated, and caught in binds—all of which he can't express directly. Until he is able to experience these directly, he won't change in a deep, meaningful way, in spite of all the sermonizing about male chauvinism and treating women as equals.

Closeness to Other Men

Daddy holds, hugs, kisses, and caresses his younger daughter but he rough and tumbles, throws around, and mock fights with his little son. A kiss on his son's lips soon sends shivers of discomfort down both their spines, so they refrain from it. Eventually a perfunctory hand-shake or a quick pat is the total permissable male-to-male physical interaction.

The boy who is openly affectionate and physically demonstrative with his brother or his male friends will feel anxious vibrations from his parents, implying doubts about his heterosexuality.

Being constantly compared with other boys in terms of achievement, teaches him that other men are his competitors and as such are also his potential enemies. "It's either me or him. We can't both win or be at the top," he may tell himself.

The need to preserve his masculine image prevents him from being transparent with other men and revealing his vulnerabilities and weaknesses. Consequently, when two men get together, the combination of underlying competitiveness, fear of homosexuality, and the need to maintain a masculine image, allow very little safe territory for involvement. It only leaves room for impersonal discussions about subjects such as automobiles, sports, politics, and business.

Throughout his early conditioning, closeness with other men was predicated on sharing a mutual enemy, whether in sports, business, or at war. As men grow older and no longer join together for these purposes, the gulf between them increases. For the average male, therefore, a close relationship with another male is at best a dim memory of high school or Army days.

Touching

"Only babies want to be held!" the young boy is told. He learns that touching is for very little children or girls. Consequently, by the time he is seven or eight he has already been conditioned to feel embarrassed and resentful if he is hugged or kissed, particularly in front of his peers. Many fathers, of course, have largely refrained from touching their sons in anything but an officious or perfunctory way after the age of two or three. "I don't want my son to grow up and become a sissy," is his rationalization.

He also learns that touching girls implies sex—you only touch if your goal is to go to bed. Adult males have profound defenses against touching; their reactions border on being phobic. They can hardly bear to be touched by other men and being touched by women is perceived as a prelude to sex. Being held and caressed for its own sake is discomforting and beyond their comprehension. The male hero images of our culture are the "untouchables"—cold, self-contained, and with no apparent need for such "sissy" behavior.

Freedom and Impulsiveness

The messages he receives as a boy that tell him not to behave like a wild animal, to "settle down," to act grown up, to control himself, teach the young adult male to fear and avoid a free-floating, spontaneous existence with many available choices. To him, being free means that he might become destructive—a bull in a china shop. He might even label himself a self-indulgent narcissist for wanting to be free. He can only enjoy freedom vicariously by identifying with fictional characters like James Bond or with the exploits of a few playboy-type swingers.

The fear of freedom drives a man to close off his options very early in life. He gets married in his early twenties, has children immediately, assumes an overload of financial responsibilities, and locks himself into a life-style with little in the way of remaining choices—long before he has even had time to really grow up and know who he is. In effect, he is building walls against freedom and impulse, which he fears will lead him into destructive, dangerous territory.

When I asked a number of men why they married and remained so, a frequently heard response was, "She has a good effect on me. She stabilizes me. She's helped me to settle down." This recurring theme reflects the male's distrust of his own ability to regulate his life and his concomitant belief in the magical powers of the woman to do that for him. In effect, these men were all marrying mother figures to whom they assigned the responsibility of making sure they behaved themselves like good boys.

Even after divorce, many men cannot seem to tolerate the freedom of a few years of unattached movement. Instead, they rush to remarry or prove that they are mature by forming another binding relationship.

Femininity

Most "straight" males would break into a cold sweat if they had to put on female clothing. While girls seem comfortable with names that sound boyish like Marty, Ronnie, or Lenny, no boy would be caught dead with or survive having a girlish name such as Sally, Sue, or Wendy. His sister could safely imitate daddy's mannerisms but his imitating of mommy is taboo. The liberation of the female has freed her almost totally to pursue and indulge in any of what was once considered traditionally masculine behavior or style. The male, however,

is still role-rigid, afraid to give expression to the female component in him. Role rigidity makes his life precarious. In a
changing world where women are increasingly taking traditionally male jobs it leaves him with few alternatives.

As a boy the messages he was given were powerful and
clear. Only sissies or "fags" play with girls. Playing house,
cooking, sewing, dressing a doll, or skipping rope would expose him to all kinds of taunts, and only the strongest could
survive and continue doing so openly.

The fear of the feminine inside of himself also tends to
make him cruel toward other men who behave in "effete"
ways. The tendency of boys to ridicule other boys who are
effeminate in their behavior and to have to posture in macho-
like behavior is all self-destructive and alienating.

"Irrational" Behavior

Silliness, clowning, being spontaneously playful, and even
laughing uninhibitedly (rather than controlled snickering) are
beyond the comfortable repertoire of typical male expression.
I am always pained when I see the embarrassed looks and
critical stares directed at a man who is letting go, clowning,
being silly, or in some way acting child-like. The unspoken
messages directed at him are, "You're making an idiot out of
yourself," or "Stop acting like an ass!" If he happens to be
elderly, the message of "No fool like an old fool!" sounds
through the room. And if he's with his wife, her discomfort is
usually plainly evident as she tries to "simmer down" her husband.

The link between being masculine and being logical, analyt-
ical, and scientific cause the male to fear the "irrational," i.e.,
anything that is not concretely visible or subject to scientific
proof. Consequently, he often lacks what is commonly referred to as "intuition," the capacity to sense and feel out a
situation and to recognize and trust his responses where the
cues are not plainly visible.

A traditional definition of male maturity involves projecting
an adult, controlled exterior with no visible childlike behavior.
Consequently, men often make boring companions. Their
tightness, self-consciousness and fear of letting go make them

overly serious and they cynically reject playfulness. About as loose as many males will allow themselves to be is to get drunk and tell "dirty" jokes or take in a porno movie.

Early admonitions that warned him not to act like a kid, not to be childish or silly, not to act crazy or like a clown lock him into a very narrow range of acceptable behavior. Self-sufficiency and strength are not seen as compatible with silliness and playfulness.

Ambiguity and Conflict

Related to his fear of the "irrational" is the fear of ambiguity. He therefore comes to need a black and white world and will buy a wrong or partial answer to relieve the anxiety associated with the grey areas, the unclear or ambiguous.

This fear of ambiguity and conflict ties in with early conditioning that pressed him to be decisive, action-oriented, logical, and clear. It is difficult to function in this style and still be accepting of vagueness and the truth of alternative possibilities.

He needs things to be good or bad, right or wrong, moral or immoral, crazy or sane, our side or their side. This attitude prevents a flexible, open approach to life. For him, there can be no twilight zones. For example, in his traditional attitude to justice, one is either innocent or guilty. Nothing in between seems tolerable. Every experience or reaction must be labeled and the truth of the existence of opposites and contradictions within the same person or life-event makes him uncomfortable.

The inability to tolerate ambiguity and conflict carries over directly to the emotional level. Consequently, the male is rigid in a relationship. It comes down to either dominate or be dominated, be in control or out of it, be strong or be vulnerable. However, he can't comfortably give play to the full dimension of his being, allowing himself to be one way at one time and some other way at another time. For as soon as he gets into forbidden territory, i.e., lets himself be dependent, it makes him uncomfortable and anxious.

Defensive Postures

It is not difficult to see why the contemporary male is sometimes referred to as a machine. Upon close examination it seems clear that few, if any feelings and expression of needs are within the socially approved definition of masculinity. Consequently, the male adopts various postures, styles, and attitudes, such as the following, to justify the fact that emotional expressiveness and survival are for him not compatible.

The Cynical Male: In his eyes all feelings are phony. His perception of himself and others is tinged with a caustic, bitter, and resigned flavor. He seems to be saying, "There ain't no way I'm ever going to get to feel and be safe in this world at the same time." So he justifies his own cynical position by labeling feelings as insincere.

The Autonomous Male: To him "feelings are weaknesses," that take him off the dead center of pure independence and only make him feel vulnerable. To the autonomous male, exposing feelings would be comparable to sticking one's Achilles heel in the face of the enemy's gun.

The Intellectualized Male: He dissects, analyzes, philosophizes, and endlessly discusses feelings, but nary a spontaneous feeling is ever emitted from him. Perhaps he even tries to "help" others to feel but his own responses are flat, detached, and impersonal. He distances himself from feelings by pouring all his own responses through the deadening filter of his intellect.

The Passive-Aggressive Male: "What do you want me to feel?" is the attitude of the passive-aggressive male. He handles his fear of feelings by non-engagement. He holes up under his shell and makes others, who may be so motivated, fight for a feeling from him. Eventually they come to leave him alone in total frustration.

The Manipulative Male: He consumes and spits up people after he has used them. He will falsely portray and mimic any feeling that he believes will get him where he wants to go. Other people's feelings are his handles, the tools he uses and the vulnerabilities he plays with in order to achieve his goal. His only feelings are of the mock variety.

The Achieving Male: "You can't eat feelings," and "Feelings are all right for later but right now they're a waste of time," is the achieving male's attitude. To the achievement-oriented male, feelings are inefficient, a luxury not connected to the vital process of survival, and in his eyes they're liable to derail him into a destructive trap. Actually, he never gets around to feeling, but maintains the illusion that he can if he so chooses.

It is very much in style today to urge men to feel. However this urging is partially reminiscent of taunting a crippled man to run. The male defenses against feeling are powerful and deep and integrally tied in with his image of himself as a man, and he is caught in roles that are the bedrock of our culture. It is unlikely that a mere act of will on his part can unlock the hurricane of repressed feelings within him. Today's man is the product of massive, defensive operations *against* feelings. These defenses are geared to protect him for survival's sake by transforming the host of powerful, socially taboo impulses, needs and feelings into acceptable male behavior. To survive and contain these repressed feelings he must detach himself increasingly from all relationships that might stimulate or provoke him into an uncontrollable response. He is comfortable primarily in denial. "I don't need you," "I'm not angry," "I don't feel like crying," etc. Because feelings are not permitted free expression the male lives in constant reaction against himself. What he is on the outside is a façade a defense *against* what he *really* is on the inside. *He controls himself by denying himself.*

Even the man who is able to release some of his emotions must always be sure to test the water first and be certain that the expression of feeling is appropriate. It may be all right to show some emotion at home, but he better be careful to keep his cool in public and especially at work. In a sense, he is forced to split his emotions, allowing some feeling to come through in only the safest places and being sure to mask his feelings in most other places.

There are many destructive consequences to the male in this situation:

1) He is vulnerable to sudden, unpredictable behavior. That is, periodically the experience of emotional starvation causes him to do "crazy" things—drinking binges, wild driving, a blatantly destructive affair, or a violent outburst, among others. All are spoutings of the inner, hidden vocano. Consequently, all of his relationships are tenuous, fragile, and explosive because his outer and inner self are so much in opposition.

2) He tends to drive those closely involved with him "crazy." That is, he denies his feelings and needs and then becomes resentful because intimates take him at face value and don't read his hidden self correctly. He ends up saying to himself, "No one really cares about me. To hell with them all."

3) The repression and unawareness of his real feelings make him prone to emotional upsets and disturbances such as depression, withdrawal, anxiety, pseudo-euphoria, etc. All of these symptoms are masking the welter of feelings that lie underneath, feelings which are blocked out of awareness. Their denial becomes the major cause of his "emotional problems."

4) The repression of feelings makes him prone to countless psychophysiological disorders. The build-up and frustration of unreleased feelings may bring on symptoms such as backaches, fatigue, headaches, bowel problems, and ulcers.

5) The defenses against feeling force him further and further away from relationships. He must keep others at a distance in order to maintain control. Consequently, he becomes increasingly lonely, alienated, numb, and with a deepening sense of futility about relationships. Only more action temporarily turns him on, but even that eventually gets run into the ground of boredom and lifelessness.

6) His inability to ask for help means that when his defenses do begin to shatter and he's caught in his own turmoil, confusion, pain, and conflict his only alternative is to withdraw even more or to numb himself with alcohol or drugs.

A man will only work to become aware of his feelings when he realizes how he is deprived of experiencing himself and the potential pleasures of being fully alive and real. The beginning of feeling will only come with the awareness of what not feeling is doing to his life. My experience as a psychotherapist has shown me, however, that one cannot simply suggest or pressure another person to feel, even if it would seem to be to their benefit. Most men have a great investment in their ability to control feelings with a concomitant fear of letting go emotionally. The male will somehow need to relearn *how* to be a feeling person.

In our culture, perhaps the safest and most facilitative way of reclaiming one's emotional self is within an individual or group therapy setting guided by a trained professional. Even here, however, one must expect that the process may be a difficult and slow one, contrary to the usual male demand that this must be quickly accomplished. Meaningful change cannot occur unless emotional experiences are fully assimilated and integrated constructively. Therefore, the male would be well advised to give himself the gift of a thorough and total experience, allowing it the time it requires and that he deserves. After all he has spent a lifetime denying his feelings. Undoing this process requires a full commitment and a constant awareness of how important this is to his survival.

5. Men In Therapy

Many men who come for psychotherapy in the midst of a painful crisis are really individuals who have fallen under the weight of what I feel is basically a male emotional dilemma. It is not so much that they are neurotic but that they are experiencing the breakthrough of feelings, impulses, needs, and conflicts that were suppressed and repressed during their early conditioning as males. These feelings were encapsulated behind powerful defenses that are now in the process of crumbling. Their emotional awareness of themselves and others had been aborted much earlier, creating critical blind spots and making them vulnerable to collapse during a crisis.

When a man's life situation is such that these verboten aspects of his emotional existence can no longer be contained by his defenses against them he arrives in the psychotherapist's office for therapy, generally in a highly agitated, anxious and/or depressed state.

ROGER R.

Age: 31
Occupation: Chemical salesman
Married: 12 years
Children: daughter—11 years,
son—8 years, son—6 years

"I guess I just went berserk. I don't know what happened to me, I just couldn't stop hitting the kid."

Roger R. came to therapy at the insistence of his wife, who threatened to leave him if he didn't. The precipitating event of their crisis took place on a Sunday afternoon. His middle son, Seth, was a hyperactive child who would get up at 6:30 every morning and go full speed ahead into late evening. They would put him to bed at 8:30 and then he would be in and out for two or three hours, going to the bathroom, asking for a story or a drink of water, pleading to watch a few minutes of television, or asking a series of questions.

The incident that caused Roger to go into a violent rage took place after a particularly hard week at work. Roger was relaxing, watching a football game while his son kept jumping all over him, asking him to play. Suddenly, Roger had what he called a "blackout." "I just grabbed Seth and started beating him and I couldn't stop. If Sylvia hadn't been around to hear the kid screaming, I might have killed him. Afterward, when she got me away and I saw the bruises on his body I started to cry. I couldn't believe what I had done."

After five therapy sessions of feeling guilty, evil, and ashamed of himself, the underlying resentments that had been brewing inside of him for years and were the long-developed cause of the Sunday incident, came pouring through. Roger had gotten married when he was nineteen because Sylvia was pregnant. "I didn't have the heart to insist she have an abortion, especially since she had already told her mother, who had told my parents. She said she loved me, wanted to be my wife and have my child. I guess I was flattered. I tried to softly reason her into an abortion and told her I'd marry her later but it didn't work. What could I do? I couldn't be a cold son of a bitch and walk away. Anyway I was a scared, middle-class kid and you don't do those things. In a way I loved her and eventually even talked myself into feeling good about becoming a father. I told myself it would make a man out of me."

His wife was only the second woman he'd ever had sex with. The first was a "back-seat job." Right after the wedding he went to work full-time, attended college in the evening, and put his remaining energies into trying to be a good father and husband.

By the time of the Sunday incident it all had been building up inside of him. "I was nothing but a well of frustration and rage. I could feel it growing everyday. Sometimes I'd be driving home wishing the house was burned down with everyone in it. Sick, isn't it? Somebody had to get my rage sooner or later. It was just a question of when."

Roger had long envied the single men he knew. He daydreamed constantly about sex. On his business trips out of town, he would go off to see a porno film. "All that did was sicken me. Here I had a wife and three kids at home and I was sitting there watching some girl blowing fifteen guys." He couldn't even pick up a girl when he was traveling because he had almost no extra money and his wife knew about every cent he spent.

He thought about leaving his wife but felt too guilty to get a divorce. "How could I abandon a very tired, very old lady?" he said. So he continued to hold it all in until that Sunday afternoon when the buried feelings just took over, all by themselves.

Roger R., like many people in our culture, got married and had children many years too soon and for many of the wrong reasons. His growth stopped when he got married. Unlike the common notion, marriage didn't mature him—it stunted him. He could no longer afford to change or to feel. He had to block everything out or it might interfere with his major goal, which was economic survival. In some senses, he was the product of a culture that tacitly condones early marriage and does not educate the male as to the heavy price he will pay for becoming strictured in this fashion.

Roger R. became a father not because he really wanted to but because he felt too guilty not to. He had the typical culturally induced male guilt reaction toward the woman; refusing to accommodate a pregnant girl was unworthy behavior. He also felt responsible for her feelings and her self-respect. The male is especially inclined to feel guilty if the woman says she loves him and wants to be the mother of his child. He also seduced himself with the notion that becoming a father would somehow validate his manhood and mature him—a typical male fantasy.

His initial resistance to getting married was manifestation of an underlying awareness that he would be giving up his growth and development. Like most middle-class men, however, he had been taught that he had to take responsibility for sexually "impulsive" behavior, if the woman so insisted. He was, in fact, legally responsible. He tried everything to fit happily into his role and continually repressed his resentful feelings until they could no longer be contained. His son finally became the target of eleven years worth of rage and frustration.

HENRY B.

Age: 39
Occupation: Owner of a boat
     salvaging company
Married: 12 years
Children: none

> "I've got those boat people by the balls. When they come begging for a part their asses are in the palm of my hand."

Henry B., a thirty-nine-year-old German immigrant, came to this country at the age of seven. Out of necessity, in order to help support his family, he started working almost immediately by helping a newspaperman unload bundles from his truck early in the morning and by delivering packages from the neighborhood butcher shop after school. His father, after a series of non-skilled jobs, got work as a welder in a shipyard, where he would often take Henry in the summer. In time Henry developed a fascination with boats and after graduating from high school took a job with a boat construction company. After doing this work for seven years, he began his own business salvaging wrecked and sunken boats. He built the business into a world-wide operation and accumulated one of the largest stocks of used, hard-to-get parts which he would then sell at a large profit.

He gloried in his success and also in his Iowa-born "all American" wife whom he married when he was twenty-seven, just as the business was beginning to become lucrative. After five years of marriage they were financially able to leave the middle-class area of town in which they lived and move to the most exclusive section. Henry admittedly felt out of place among the wealthy because he still considered himself a blue-collar person. He always had communicated well with construction workers and other skilled laborers. However, he got vicarious pleasure knowing that his wife was enjoying the status and was thriving as part of the local "society."

When he came into therapy his reasons for being there were at first very vague. He spoke of being "too nervous" and wanting to learn how to relax. He spent the better part of the first five sessions bragging about his success, often in hostile tones. "I'm the top man in this business. They come to me on my terms, or else. If they don't like my prices they can shove it. I've paid plenty of dues to get where I am," he said.

His therapist confronted Henry. "You're not paying me all of this money to brag about your accomplishments, are you?"

Henry reddened, became evasive, then finally said, "Ah, fuck it, I might as well tell you now." Then he revealed that in the last five years he had become homosexual, active in the bathrooms of parks and at train stations, primarily when he was out of town. He decided to seek help after he had just missed being arrested by a policeman in plainclothes. He managed to talk his way out of it but the incident terrified him. He envisioned his whole life going up in smoke.

His homosexual feelings only had begun to obsess him after he had become successful. Up until then he had an occasional homosexual fantasy, but suppressed it by working hard, competing, and "making it." When he finally allowed himself to experience his strong sexual desires for men he was too afraid to go to gay bars or to try and meet gays at other places because he feared being recognized.

Henry said it hadn't affected his marriage because his wife didn't seem to mind the fact that they seldom had sex. When they did he would fantasize male partners. She seemed content just being a part of the active social scene and interpreted his general lack of sexual interest as being due to overwork. As Henry continued talking about this he realized he was deeply resentful about her luxuriating in that style of life. "I really hate living in that part of town. At least before I had someone to talk to. Now it's all a bullshit trip with some wealthy WASPS," he admitted.

Henry B. typified many upwardly mobile men who end up living in wealthy surroundings in which they are basically unhappy and have little in common with their neighbors. Driven to prove themselves, to please their wives, and impress their friends they end up uncomfortable and isolated in a setting which is not for them.

In many ways, Henry's acting out is an example of how many success-oriented men end up doing something self-destructive in an unconscious attempt to free themselves from an increasingly unreal, unsatisfying life. Perhaps they flagrantly have an affair, begin drinking heavily, become illegally manipulative in business, begin ignoring or forgetting important commitments, etc., all in an unconscious wish to be released from a painful situation that they are not consciously capable of walking away from. In Henry's case the setting in which he chose to indulge his homosexual impulses was almost guaranteed to result in disaster. In one sense Henry was trying to destroy a life he had built and which had become sterile and deadening.

Henry's attitude toward his competitors symbolizes the possible connection in our culture between hostile, cut-throat behavior in business and sublimated male homosexuality. Men in business insult each other by calling each other "assholes," often speak of having each other "by the balls," giving it to each other "up the ass" and "screwing" or "being screwed" by a competitor. Henry's homosexual behavior didn't emerge overtly until *after* he had made it in business, when he no longer needed to sublimate his homosexuality into hostile, competitive behavior.

In a sense the culture's hostile attitude toward the expression of the feminine in men may have a direct relationship to the severe alienation and distrust that exists among them, most graphically seen in the more competitive areas such as business. These cut-throat attitudes of men can be seen as a reaction *against* the culturally fearsome, threatening impulse to be close with males. These attitudes push the male into super-macho behavior and produce a dread of closeness with other men.

STEVEN L.

Age: 26
Occupation: Tennis instructor
Marital Status: Single

". . . I've screwed all these chicks and I can't even remember most of their names."

Steven L. was an attractive, darkly complexioned, athletically built male. He had been a physical education major in college and a member of the tennis team. After graduation he took a job at a newly built tennis club housed in a large singles complex. There he was constantly meeting girls on the courts, as well as at parties and at singles bars. He came for therapy after having been to bed with a series of girls, experiences that left him with a deepening sense of loneliness and boredom. "I feel like I've had ten thousand dates and I'm living in a sea of bodies. Every time I score I flash in my head how many I've made."

For several years Steven had even thrived on what he called "traffic jams." He would make as many as three dates on the same day—beginning in late afternoon, followed by one at nine o'clock, and ending up at another girl's apartment at midnight. He found he had less and less to say to his dates. It seemed like an endless succession of going for a drink or dinner, maybe to a movie and then home to bed. He was bored and angry with his girl friends for going along passively with whatever he suggested. "They never let me know where they're at. I don't know what they really like or don't like or even who they are. They just kind of go along. Sometimes I feel like saying to them, 'You drive and I'll sit and watch the damn scenery. You decide where to go and what to do.' Even when we fuck they don't tell me what turns them on. They're so busy pleasing me that I think most of the time they're bullshitting me and themselves with their pretenses at being turned on." Though Steve was angry at the passivity of his dates he admitted that he didn't like girls who were "too aggressive" either. If he sensed that they were pushy he wouldn't date them at all.

While claiming that he wanted a more meaningful relationship he knew he also was defeating himself. Though he was invariably critical of little things about his dates, the way they dressed, smelled, talked or moved, he would never tell them what about them he didn't like. He would just silently cross them off the list. He saw his reason as being that he didn't want to hurt them. The deeper reason came out in one session when he said, "I don't tell them because I really don't want them to change for me. How would I know whether they're not just manipulating me by changing to please me. Later when they're more secure they'll always go back to the old patterns anyway."

Though he was seemingly very aggressive with women he realized he would always wait for a sign that they found him attractive before he would approach one. Rarely would he pursue a girl he was attracted to if she seemed indifferent, and once a girl had refused a date he would never ask a second time. "I hate selling anything—including myself," he said.

Though he was proud of being a tennis instructor he felt that the girls he dated were attracted to him largely because of his image and didn't know or seem to care who he really was. Yet he recognized that he set it up that way by getting the fact that he was a tennis instructor into the conversation on the first date and by mainly dating girls he met on the tennis courts.

Steven was a product of the contradictory male conditioning which places him in a no-win conflict by reinforcing him for "scoring" and then making him feel guilty about it, not allowing him to really enjoy it by labeling his behavior as "shallow," or indicating to him that it comes from a Don Juan sense of sexual insecurity and is a reflection of his inability to relate "meaningfully." In Steven's case he wasn't able to enjoy sexual experiences for their own sake nor could he accept alternatives such as a monogamous relationship or even no sex at all.

Again, typical of male conditioning, Steven was afraid of leveling about his negative feelings with his dates lest he hurt their feelings. The male is taught to treat women non-aggressively and to view them as fragile. This prevents a relationship from building on an emotionally real basis. Furthermore, the male fear of being manipulated by a woman, who might temporarily change to please him, is also a result of his inability to properly read the difference between a genuine and a manipulative response. This stems, in part, from his conditioned fear of trusting his own responses and his tendency to call himself "hostile" if he confronts a woman immediately, when he feels a response is not genuine.

While forced into imagining himself as Steven did by telling his dates he was a tennis instructor (in order to be found attractive), the male becomes a victim of that same process. That is, he struggles to become "somebody" and after he does he experiences that deep sense of loneliness that comes from feeling compelled to stay in a role to be attractive, all the while realizing that he is not being recognized or loved for who and what he really is.

While superficially the pursuers, most males have never developed rejection tolerance in their relations with women. Unconsciously this drives them toward those women who they sense already find them attractive. While it is reassuring to be sought after, there is at the same time an underlying, frustrating realization that in important ways the choice in the relationship was not really his.

Finally, Steven had the traditional male resistance against being passive in the relationship with women. Consequently, he tended to shy away from the assertive woman and be attracted to the more passive "feminine" woman, only to feel resentful because he was repeatedly in a lopsided, repetitive interaction in which he always felt compelled to be the dominant one.

LEONARD S.

> Age: 67
> Occupation: Retired teacher
> Married: 34 years
> Children: son—31 years
> daughter—28 years

"He keeps making little sex jokes around the young girls. He must be getting senile and I'm worried about him."

Leonard S. was referred for therapy by his physician at the repeated urging of his wife, Jenny, who made the appointment for him because Leonard refused to do it himself. Over the phone she explained with concern that he seemed to be acting inappropriately, was staring incessantly at young girls and would often make remarks that embarrassed her and the family. Jenny, a beautiful woman with a stern, "practical" look and snow white hair tied in a bun, came to the therapy session with Leonard, a robust, vital-looking grey-haired man. Jenny did most of the talking initially while Leonard sat quietly, looking alternately embarrassed and irritated. Even though she acknowledged that Leonard was a healthy man she was convinced that he must have had a lot of those "little strokes" she had read about in a doctor's newspaper column, "the kind that don't give you a real stroke but damage your brain."

"I don't understand what's happening to him," she said. "In the last two years he's started to talk to all the young hippies in the park. When we're walking in the streets he stares at the young girls with no bras and their nipples showing through. He looks as if his eyes are going to pop out of his head. The latest thing is that he walks by the nude beach near our home all the time and two weeks ago he wanted to take all his clothes off. He would have if I hadn't stopped him." She also complained that Leonard wasn't interested in opera anymore, the way he used to be. Instead he would stand fixated, listening to the young people at the beach playing rock music.

Jenny exploded in rage when Leonard finally spoke and said, "There's nothing wrong with me at all. Our friends are boring—you want me to play shuffleboard or chess all day like they do." Jenny interrupted him immediately, asking him accusingly what he could possibly get out of talking to young people. "They don't know anything. They're babies. They're confused enough and instead of helping them you're trying to act like them."

Jenny was particularly embarrassed about Leonard's long walks alone in the evening. Occasionally he would meet young teenage girls, get in a discussion with them, charm them, and invite them over to the house for coffee. Once a couple of them came because they thought he was "adorable." This incident embarrassed Jenny so much that she couldn't continue talking about it. In a fit of intensifying irritation she blurted out that it would be better if Leonard were dead rather than going around making a fool of himself. She quickly apologized and explained that she really didn't mean it that way. "After you've been a teacher and a respected man all these years and everybody knows us, I can't understand it. You don't see any other men your age making an idiot out of themselves. I'm ashamed that our grandchildren might run into you and see you acting this way." Leonard sat quietly as Jenny kept looking to the therapist for some support for her belief that Leonard had a "brain problem." When this was not forthcoming and when the therapist instead urged Leonard to share his feelings and to confront Jenny, she became uncomfortable and asked if the hour was over yet.

The reaction to Leonard's behavior, one that typifies the reaction older men in our culture generally get when they evince an interest in younger girls, is a reflection of the culture's rigid notions of "age-appropriate" behavior.

Elderly men are supposed to find their satisfactions among their peers—even if such involvements are boring and unfulfilling to them—and often labeled "dirty old men" and "lechers" for staring at and enjoying, even though usually vicariously, younger girls. It seems to be particularly threatening to the elderly man's family who become uncomfortable, distressed, and confused if he steps out of his expected role of "grandpa."

An exception to this is when the elderly man happens to be powerful, wealthy and/or of high status. In that case there seems to be more social tolerance. In other instances however, the older man is vulnerable to looks of embarrassment and resentment from others and mutterings of "no fool like an old fool" when he tries to enjoy himself with younger girls.

It is particularly distressing if the younger girls reciprocate the interest, even if only in a playful, perhaps teasing way. Immediately others want to "protect" the older man from himself. Should he be behaving in an un-self-conscious spontaneous way the assumption is that he is acting inappropriately rather than reflecting a rebirth of male vitality and excitement.

The family's anxiety about his behavior reflects their needs to cast him into a predictable, rigid, depressing role that suits their needs, not his. Clearly it seems that they are more comfortable being "helpful" and "concerned" over his illnesses and aging debilities, than in sharing with him the joys of his spontaneity and renewed sexual interest and curiosity.

WARREN P.

Age: 30
Occupation: Manager of a sporting
  goods store
Marital Status: Separated
Children: None

"I was totally committed to her. Isn't that what you psychotherapists always say is supposed to make a good relationship?"

Warren P. came for therapy because his twenty-seven-year-old, finely featured red-haired wife was dissatisfied with their sex life. Though he himself said he had no complaints, was always turned on by her, he was willing, he said, to help her in her "battle" to overcome her frigidity. This was only one in a long series of "battles" Warren engaged in to prove his devotion and commitment to his wife. With tears in his eyes he described his feelings about her. "It's almost like I am the gardener and she's the seed. It satisfies me just to help her to grow and to blossom."

That was, in many ways, the essence of their five-year relationship. When he and his wife, Jackie, first met he was a graduate student in marine biology, planning a career in underwater research. With a superb talent for deep-sea diving he eventually hoped to become part of a team that would live for stretches of time under water exploring the bottom of the ocean.

On their first date Jackie seemed to be extremely shy and vulnerable. To Warren this was the epitome of femininity. "She wasn't pushy like the other women I'd been dating. She had a quality of fragility, or helplessness—a kind of sensitivity that really turned me on. I saw a great potential in her to become a fantastic woman and I remember telling myself that if all I ever did in life was to help her achieve her potential I would be more than satisfied. I wasn't worried about my career— those kind of ego trips weren't important to me. She was all that really mattered."

A year after he met her they married and he took a job managing a shop that sold and repaired diving equipment. When he wasn't working, he dedicated himself to Jackie. He encouraged her to go to college part-time. "I felt she was too sensitive to go full-time. I didn't want her to get crushed by the education machine. Still I knew it was important for her to feel better about herself since she only had a high school degree and I had graduate credits." In the evenings he would help her write term papers.

That was only one of the many ways he tried to help her during the next four years. For example, one day when he saw her dancing around the apartment he decided that she had undeveloped talent. So he encouraged her to enroll in a modern dance class and told her that if she studied he was sure she eventually would be discovered.

He also accompanied her to the dentist to get her teeth capped and to diet doctors to help her with her weight control problem. Because she was small breasted he even suggested the possibility of implant surgery but she was scared. Saturdays he would often take her clothes shopping, even though their money situation was tight. "It felt good to love somebody more than myself for a change," he said. "It made me feel 'pure' inside."

Meanwhile he let his own interests go. He gave up his hobby of underwater photography because there wasn't enough money for materials. He became overweight because he didn't have time to work out, and he gave up most of his close friendships because there just wasn't enough time to be with them and he felt that his wife really needed him more and that gave him satisfaction.

Originally when she complained of being unable to respond to him sexually he even gave her permission to have affairs during the day, while he was at work. "I felt the experience might help her and I was so sure that she loved and depended on me that it didn't threaten me." When that didn't help their sex life he agreed to try sex therapy with her.

Sex therapy procedures eventually led to discussions about other things with the therapist. Warren was severely stunned during one session when Jackie, in quiet, icy tones told him that she hated him for trying to make her over. She accused him of being a boring person and made disparaging comments about the fact that he had dropped out of school and was only working in a diving gear store when he could have made something of himself. Rage came pouring from his wife when she sarcastically insulted him for giving her permission to have relations with other men. "The guys I slept with told me they thought you were an idiot and that if I was their woman they'd never let me do it."

Warren felt betrayed and hurt by her outburst but consoled himself by thinking, "She's getting in touch with her anger and that'll help her grow more." But just when she seemed to get to the point where she was becoming a total person and he was ready to do something for himself, she announced that she was leaving. She had fallen in love with a man, she said, "Who doesn't take shit from me, who doesn't treat me like his child, who accepts me for what I am and who would kill me if I even looked at another man!"

Warren was immobilized for months, crying and waiting for her to "come to her senses" and return home. "Nobody'll ever love her the way that I did. She'll get crushed. She'll find out."

Warren was an extreme example of the male "blind spot" in regard to the illusion of "femininity"—the need to search out and maintain a fantasy of the "real" woman as fragile, vulnerable, and in need of protection and guidance. Often the male proceeds in some fashion to dedicate himself to his woman's well-being, growth, and fulfillment. This partially reflects the male fear of being aggressive toward the woman. His defenses against these feelings operate in such a way as to transform the aggression in him into the more socially acceptable impulse to be super protective of her.

It also reflects the male's self-hate, his tendency to see himself as selfish and insensitive. He attempts to overcome these feelings by depriving himself in order to please her. When he's "in love" he selflessly can put himself second and feel righteous denying his own needs and aborting his own development in favor of hers.

Warren's behavior also reflected the male need to believe in the existence of the aggressionless female. Because her aggression does not manifest itself in the more direct forms typical of the male he believes it doesn't exist at all in women, particularly in his. He is unable to see her aggression emerging in countless indirect ways—including that of exerting powerful manipulative control through her reactions of "helplessness" and "fragility." When her anger and rage finally emerge directly at some later point, as it eventually did with Jackie, he is surprised, overwhelmed, and disbelieving. He is liable to feel that he deserved it and must have pushed her to an extreme to get her to this point or that she was just temporarily not herself.

The male is also vulnerable in the male-female relationship because he denies his own dependency needs. Unconsciously, he tends to obtain his dependency satisfactions vicariously and indirectly by allowing the woman to depend on him. In a sense, she is acting out his unexpressed, starved part and he is gaining gratification indirectly. He continues to nurture the illusion that dependency is a one-way street until the relationship is threatened or she leaves him. Then, he frequently discovers that in truth he was the more deeply dependent one. This ties in directly with the male tendency to relate to his female intimate as a child, only to discover that she is, in many critical ways, less vulnerable and childlike than he is.

ANTHONY S.

Age: 51
Occupation: Record producer
Marital Status: Divorced
Children: son—16 years,
        daughter—13 years, daughter—11 years

"I'm big daddy to these tennyboppers. I buy them things and they'll do anything for me—go down on me in the recording booth—if that's what I want."

Anthony S., a New York-born high school drop-out was a self-made man. He began his working life doing menial jobs in the garment center. While there he became friendly with some blacks who turned him on to "soul music"—the music of the black blues musicians. He was drawn to this kind of music because of a deep sense of empathy for the underdog and anger and resentment at the "smug, apathetic, privileged segment of the population."

He decided that his life mission would be to bring this beautiful and moving music to the attention of white people. So he formed a partnership with his best friend, a neighborhood buddy of his from the time he was eleven. Together they searched for undiscovered talent in small clubs in Harlem, the south side of Chicago, and cities down South. His partner would take care of the business aspects while Anthony would take care of the artistic part—recording the artists.

While he started the record company with the noble intention of making a social contribution by helping unknown musicians gain recognition, his attitude slowly began to change. "I'm never going to make it unless I accept the realities of this business and stop playing Florence Nightingale," he began to tell himself. His business approach became increasingly cutthroat. He began to draw up contracts with new artists that were totally exploitive—long-term contracts that gave him all the options and most of the money and offered the artist almost no protection or advantages. He rationalized this to himself saying, "I'm taking all the risks to expose these guys. They'll make their money in live performances."

He initially went into business out of the love of music. But he became increasingly preoccupied with money and power and eventually hired others to handle the actual musical end that he once had loved. He was dissatisfied with his partner's "namby pamby" approach to business and after working together for sixteen years these best friends were no longer speaking to each other. Each came to feel the other was trying to rip him off. They got into a protracted fight which caused the business to fall apart, and they eventually went bankrupt.

By now Anthony was married with three children. His wife, an upper-class Southern belle, deeply resented it when her husband, in his desperation to make money and continue their life-style, went into the business of illegally bootlegging records. He would tape albums released by major companies, press records, and sell them "underground" to record stores or by advertising on small television stations around the country.

Anthony finally came into therapy on referral from his urologist. He had become impotent a year ago. His wife, who had become socially embarrassed by his business activities, moved back to her home town in Georgia with their children. She withheld the children from him so he was fighting her in court for custody. He was now deeply in debt and becoming desperate about his disintegrating life. He also was now almost a hundred pounds overweight.

During his first session of therapy he was smooth and guarded in manner and talked in raspy tones. He was clearly embarrassed to be there. "Therapy is for women who want somebody to listen to them cry," he said. He had begged his urologist to give him injections or even an operation to restore his potency. However, he was told that it wouldn't work. In his mind, an operation or injections was a more "masculine" way to approach his problem than by talking about feelings.

He seemed to be gasping for breath as he puffed on his cigarettes and spoke: "I had it made. I came up from nowhere. Then all of a sudden it became a nightmare. My partner was out to screw me and I was screwing him back. The black musicians I once had loved and helped were starting to hate my guts. My wife who I thought would always be in my corner couldn't handle it when I went broke and was trying to earn some money bootlegging records. I tried to get a regular, straight job but as soon as they found out how old I was they turned into icebergs. So I went into the bootleg business to help pay the bills and she left with the kids. Our relationship wasn't going well anyway. I couldn't get an erection with her for over a year. I guess she just got fed up. Now I'm back in the record business surrounded by these tennyboppers. Getting caught for bootlegging doesn't scare me but one of these days I'm liable to have a rape charge laid on me and I might land in jail and they'll throw away the key."

Though he had started out his life with good intentions, twenty-five years later everything was destroyed—his love for music, his friendship, his family. "Something went wrong," he acknowledged.

Anthony's situation demonstrates how the male's drive for success can progressively destroy the intrinsic motivating joys of the original endeavor. In Anthony's case his love of music was completely suffocated in the process of meeting the "realities" of business and competition. His experience was not an exception. It is equally common among many doctors, attorneys, college professors, craftsmen, or artists. The original positive motivations and the satisfaction and pleasure they get from their work more often than not progressively deteriorates into a cynical grabbing for money, security, status, and power.

The drive for financial survival typically has a tendency to erode the friendships between men, producing deep distrust and progressively alienating them from each other. In Anthony's case he eventually alienated himself from his best friend and from the musicians for whom he originally had a genuine affection.

In the process of trying to maintain a high economic level the male also often becomes progressively alienated from his family. This has a particularly bitter impact in light of the common male illusion that he is doing it all for his wife and children. When they leave him or hold him in contempt for it, it is a particularly painful experience.

Anthony's weight problem, resulting from constant nervous eating, and his potentially self-destructive sexual involvement with very young girls can be seen partially as a form of psychological regression—an unconscious wish to destroy a self-defeating life-style coupled with a hunger to experience some

primal, intrinsically satisfying pleasures like eating and feeling
young and spontaneously sexual. In a way, it can be seen as a
wish to be a boy again, to start all over in a world of more
immediate, genuinely satisfying pleasures.

In spite of all the devastation of his life, Anthony resisted
the notion of psychotherapeutic help to the very end. To him,
talking about feelings was embarrassing—a "woman's thing."
He would have much preferred a more medical approach—an
injection or even surgery if such existed. Again Anthony was
only an extreme case of the male propensity to resist asking
for help within a relationship and his great embarrassment
over having to explore feelings and acknowledge their importance in the creation of the circumstances of his life. The
themes in Anthony's life were not unusual—only a bit more
extreme than in most men's lives.

GERALD B.

> Age: 41
> Occupation: Accountant
> Married: 17 years
> Children: daughter—16 years,
>   son—13 years

"I feel like I'm surrounded by an invisible shield.
I'm screaming for attention but nobody hears me."

Gerald B., short, slightly built and with greying hair, lived
with his wife and two children in the suburbs of a large midwestern city. He drove forty-five minutes each day to get to
his job with a large trucking company located in the center of
town.

Like most adult males he came to therapy only when he
was almost at the bottom. During the first session he described
himself as a "work-aholic." He felt numb, depressed, and totally isolated. Both at work and at home he said he felt as if he
were invisible. His relationship with his wife, once pleasurable
and satisfying, had become increasingly mechanical and repetitive. They had gradually stopped doing the things that they
used to enjoy doing together—traveling, going out for dinner,
playing tennis, and reading to each other.

Their social life with neighbors and old-time friends was all
but dead, except for an occasional formal function such as a

company barbecue, a neighborhood political meeting or a parents' meeting at the school. Early in the marriage, his wife had criticized his sloppiness in dress, the way he sat on people's sofas, his dinner manners, and his tendency to use "dirty" words. Sometimes he would drink too much and get "silly" and this would embarrass her. Consequently, going out became too painful for her and too boring for him. So they stopped it altogether.

Their home life was role rigid. He played the part of good provider and stable father. She played the role of efficient housekeeper and protective mother. He barely related to the children anymore because they had fought over their differing child-rearing attitudes and he had decided he was being too selfish. His job was his turf and the home was hers.

Consequently, he became increasingly passive at home, fading progressively into the background. His relationship to the children consisted mainly of chauffering them occasionally and giving them money. He'd barely even get an acknowledgment when he came home from work in the evenings. It was none of this "Daddy's home! Daddy's here!" he had heard in his home as a child.

His sex life with his wife Gloria, a virgin when they married, was never very adventurous to begin with and was now perfunctory. Once every few weeks they would "do it," always in the same position, always quickly, and with no display of feelings. For a while, he had tried reading and showing her "how to" books on sex. He would bring her surprise gifts to try to breathe some new life into the relationship, but nothing succeeded. He soft-pedalled the open assertion of his sexual needs because he didn't want her to think he was "horny" or an "animal." He eventually gave up trying to turn her on and would masturbate in the bathroom after she'd fallen asleep.

He had always taken his work very seriously and put most of his energies into it—so seriously, in fact, that he'd often work straight through his coffee breaks and eat his lunch out of a brown paper bag at his desk. He never learned to play what he called the "smile and handshake" game. Others began to see him as not wanting to be bothered with them and he could hardly get himself to call someone up and ask them for lunch, because he was sure they thought him as boring and didn't like him. Besides, he had blown it several times in the past by totally forgetting that he had arranged a lunch date.

Consequently, at the office his style was to work constantly and try to please by being available to others who needed his help. It seemed to him that the only time anyone approached him was when they wanted something. Though he resented it, he felt stuck. What could he really do about it?

He had been a great believer in the virtues and rewards of hard work and moral living. Now it seemed to him that there were no payoffs in it at all. His children were almost grown and he was a stranger to them. His relationship with his wife was stagnant and rigid. While he used to fantasize and get erections looking at the braless secretaries, that wasn't turning him on anymore either.

The thought of suicide no longer appalled or frightened him. In fact, he told his therapist during the first session that it was the only consoling feature in his life.

Like most men, Gerald B. had been brought up learning the necessity and importance of throwing his energies into his work. He was so committed to the virtues of responsibility and achieving security that he gradually distanced himself from friends, co-workers, and his family and gave up on the possibility of gratification of any other needs. In his diligence and his compulsion to work hard in order to fulfill his role as competent provider he boxed himself into a world without people. Like many men who isolate themselves in this way he had always been busy working—or fighting his way home through traffic to fulfill his role as dutiful and ever-present father. Even though he was passive at home he would have felt guilty not being there every evening.

He couldn't recognize his own anger at being so isolated at home and at work. Instead, he concluded that there was something wrong with him—he was some kind of pariah, unlikeable though he honestly couldn't understand why. He tried so hard and gave everybody all he had. What more could he do, he wondered.

As a typically closed male he could only surmise what others felt about him. He would never dare ask them directly, nor would he share his own feelings about them. He could never bring himself to tell someone whether he liked or disliked them. This is typical of the male fear of openly sharing feelings in a personal way with others.

Like many men, he gave up participating actively and asserting himself in decisions about child-rearing and home life and assumed an increasingly passive role. Like many other men he typically felt guilty because he was "privileged" to work and he felt, therefore, that his wife should be entitled to control her arena—the home. Besides, again in male fashion, he felt that women really did know best about raising children and he assumed that his influence would only be obstructive. He had the typically despairing sense of being a transparent meal ticket and nothing more.

The conditioned male fear of aggression toward a woman also severely affected his relationship with his wife. She was his only intimate in the world and as the years went by he became increasingly afraid that if he confronted her with his resentment and discontent he might lose her and be totally alone. He also could never bring himself to talk directly about sex because she was a "good woman." In spite of what he had read about the so-called liberalization of sex he felt it was too late for them. He made do with what little there was and filled in the spaces with masturbation.

His sensitivity to her criticism about his social manners and appearance, and the feeling that she might be right, caused him to withdraw. Like most men he didn't trust his own social responses and sensed it was wrong just to be himself when he was at other people's homes or even at his own home when company was over. Since he got no pleasure out of the alternative, which was superficial party chatter, there was no social life. Where he had had many male friends before he was married, as time passed, because of his heavy involvement with work and his sense of responsibility toward his family, he no longer had any close male relationships.

Gerald B. felt there was nothing of meaning left in his life. He felt betrayed by life because he had done everything he had learned a man should do and had come up with a zero.

PHILIP F.

Age: 31
Occupation: Electrical contractor
Marital Status: Separated
Children: son—3 years

"I'll do anything to get her back. Please tell me how to change."

Philip F. found out by accident that his wife, Cindy, was having an affair. When he confronted her he was surprised that she didn't even deny it. Instead she told him that she couldn't take being a mother and a wife anymore and thought that she was on the verge of a nervous breakdown. She claimed that she wasn't in love with the other man but had to get away for awhile "to think things over." Philip would ask her pleadingly if she still loved him and her answer would be, "I really don't know how I feel right now. I'm too confused." Philip would search out any sign, a look, a word that he could interpret as indicating that she still loved him.

Philip F. came for therapy trembling and shaking. He listed all the horrible things about himself—self-accusations that originally had been accusations directed at him by his wife. He was too detached, too compulsive in his work, too selfish, too narcissistic. He pleaded for ways to change that might get her back.

He began: "Five years ago I left my first wife to be with Cindy after I'd known her less than three weeks. She had the magic. She'd always say the exactly right thing at the right time. She was beautiful and sexy. She'd tell me I made her whole body tingle and I was the first man who turned her on completely. Over and over she'd say, 'Baby I love you so much.'

"I guess I knew in my guts that it was too good, too unreal to last. Guys were always staring at her and I knew she was loving it. Her favorite songs were always about living and loving now and forgetting about tomorrow. And I had to do almost all of the talking. She'd just sit and give me these adoring looks and then say something that made me feel like the strongest, most beautiful, together guy in the world.

"But still something was wrong. She'd tell me she'd meet me at seven and show up at nine, or she'd ask me to call her from work at a certain time and she wouldn't be there. She always had a good excuse and teased me for being compulsive. I had this feeling though that whatever was in front of her, that's what got her complete attention."

The shocker came three weeks after Cindy had moved out without giving Philip her address. They met for dinner one evening and got to talking about sex. Cindy confessed that she had never, even at the beginning, had an orgasm with him. All the while he had believed he was turning her on incredibly.

Then she told him she felt that having had a baby was a mistake and that she wanted Philip to keep the baby. This tore Philip apart. It was she who had originally wanted the child and not him. He only agreed because he thought it was important to her and now she wanted to walk away from it all.

For two months after that Philip alternated between deep despair, guilt, and murderous rage. At one point he wanted to kill her and her boyfriend. In spite of these feelings, even though he had the baby and now she was living with another man he continued to send her support money every month. "I wanted her to know that I understand she's in trouble and I won't abandon her." He hung onto the belief that it was all a part of an emotional breakdown and that she'd pull out of it and come back to him.

In therapy, Philip was able to cry when he remembered how she used to hold on to him, caressing him and calling him, "Baby, baby," and how special she made him feel. "It was like dope and I was addicted. Just having her touch me made me feel like Superman." But when the therapist asked Philip to describe Cindy as a person Philip could only do so in very vague terms. She was really a mystery and a shadow to him.

"Mainly she just listened to me and sent out all of these love vibes. But she never talked about herself very much."

Cindy kept him hanging on for over a year. Every time he'd decide never to see her again, she would call and say she missed him and that she knew how painful it must be for him. She'd come over occasionally and go to bed with him and go home. Then he wouldn't hear from her again for days or weeks. She'd raise his hopes by telling him how bad her new relationship was and that it really was sexless. Philip would believe her, even though he knew otherwise. Somehow she always was able to say what he needed to hear at the right time. He knew that she did this but he couldn't help believing her anyway. He wanted to believe her.

He'd ask her to come back home and she'd tell him she wasn't ready yet. She needed more time to think. And this was a year and a half after she'd originally left him to "think" for a little while.

Eventually, Philip began to see how he was using therapy not to change himself but to find ways to get back to her and also to let her know that if she came back he'd be a new man.

Consequently, he was hardly changing at all. He was just holding on to the status quo and waiting. She gave him an occasional love crumb and he held onto the fantasy that she'd eventually come to her senses. He tried dating other girls but his thoughts always drifted back to her.

Philip exemplified a surprisingly common male propensity. He had a fixation and fascination with a rejecting female. And it seems the more he is rejected, the harder he clings and the more "in love" he perceives himself as being.

This phenomenon seems to have two aspects to it. On one level it feeds into the male excitement over a challenge. At the same time the woman may also have a way of "adoring" that feeds into the male need to believe in the "magic woman," the female who recognizes the superman in him and worships him for it. This need causes him to have a blind spot for this kind of woman and causes him to believe the unbelievable.

It also feeds into his fantasy of omnipotence—the tendency to so distort his perception of the female that he firmly believes that she couldn't possibly care for anybody else and if she did it would only be because she was trying to punish him.

Philip also personifies the not unusual male ignorance about female sexuality that makes him vulnerable to conning himself into believing she is having super orgasms when she is really only faking her responses. This is just one example of the overall male inability to read the female correctly. When Cindy said she wanted a baby, even though Philip didn't want one, he came to feel that she knew best, that her maternal needs had to be fulfilled so he went along with it. He wanted to show her he loved her. The shock came when he discovered that his original resistance to having a child was correct and that, contrary to his fantasy about how maternal his wife was, she didn't really enjoy being a mother.

Because of his need to feel he is totally central, he is unable to read the woman he is fixated on and is therefore shocked when he discovers she's having an affair. Even then he often tends to disbelieve her and to imagine that she's only saying this to excite or provoke him and that she couldn't really love another man.

Finally, Philip is typical of the male approach to therapy in these situations when an important relationship is breaking down. He comes looking for ways to change in order to get his woman back rather than to change for his own growth as a person.

Many of the so-called emotional problems of a man are actually growth crises. They are cracks in his defenses created by the persistent pressure of his underlying emotional core. These defenses prevented him from seeing himself or others realistically as total people. He frequently breaks down at a period in life where the prospects of real change are frightening for he already has invested too heavily in his illusions to be open to growth and change.

The thrust of the "help" he often gets from relatives and well-meaning friends is of the band-aid variety. He will be encouraged to overcome or control his symptoms or, in patchwork style, to put back the pieces as close to the way they were before as possible, instead of learning to understand the symptoms as representing an inner demand for a new emotional totality. The male in our culture must be coached to listen respectfully to these crises as signaling the beginning of a rebirth into full personhood. He should be taught to celebrate his crises for the important truths that they are revealing and the reawakening which they portend.

6. Impossible Binds

The male in our culture finds himself in countless "damned if you do, damned if you don't" no-win binds. He is constantly being affected by gross inconsistencies—between what he had been taught was "masculine" behavior as a boy and what is expected of him as an adult; between inner needs and social pressures; and between contradictory expectations in the many roles he has to play. He is psychologically fragmented by these many contradictory demands. For survival's sake, he is literally forced into functioning in a machine-like, emotionally detached, and extremely repressed way. In other words, the traditional male facade—cool, detached, controlled, guarded, and disengaged—is a protective mechanism that allows him to respond simply to external cues or inputs, like a programmed computer, rather than having to wrestle with constant conflict and ambiguity.

The first step in coping with this phenomenon is open recognition and acknowledgment of these binds.

The Gender Bind

The male child is raised with a strong feminine imprint. His deepest emotional relationships and some of his most profound influences are mother, grandmother, and teacher, who is more often than not a woman. Father, very likely, is a background figure, home for relatively short periods of time during the week and frequently preoccupied and minimally involved when he is around. The young boy is therefore being conditioned by the female identity much of the time. As if by magic, by the time he reaches the age of five or six he is expected to become "all boy." The heavy female component to his identity must be repressed. To express it, or to behave in a feminine way, is to open himself up to derisive inferences, ridicule, and hostile name-calling such as "sissy" and "fag."

To survive in this culture, therefore, the male must disown and deny a major portion of his deepest identification. He does this through a defense psychologists call reaction formation, a form of going to the opposite extreme. This results in a macho style of relating—the supermale posture. The price is rigid, overcontrolling of emotions and a denial of a part of himself.

Either way he loses: If he is in touch with and expressive of his feminine component he may be subject to great feelings of anxiety and humiliation. If he successfully manages to repress, disown, and deny this critical part of himself he will have to live as an incomplete person, alienated from an important part of himself and consequently susceptible to emotional and interpersonal rigidity and numerous psychological and psychophysiological problems that result from this repression.

The Kinetic Bind

As a young boy he will be encouraged and praised for being movement-oriented, active, boisterous, playful and for using his physical strength and agility. That will define him as a "real boy." However, in order to be successful in school and later on in the professional white collar, middle-class occupations he will have to repress that physicalness. For example, he will have to sit still for long stretches of time and to be passive and physically inactive when he feels the need for being just the opposite. Perhaps he will begin to smoke, drink coffee constantly, use alcohol or stuff himself with food in order to distract and numb himself sufficiently so that being confined and caged will be more tolerable.

Either way he loses: If he stays in touch with and is expressive of his need to be physically active and to move and use his body he may be less successful in school and at work. He will been seen as "restless," a behavior problem, poorly disciplined, hyperactive, maladjusted, etc. On the other hand, if he becomes comfortably able to conform, it will probably be at the price of denying the existence and needs of his body. As a result he will tend to become a prototype of the typical middle-aged male who has manifested a drastic physical decline in a relatively short period of time after his youth.

The Feeling Bind

Throughout his life, if he expresses his feelings openly and readily cries, screams, behaves sensually, etc., he may be viewed as "unstable" or "neurotic." If he controls his feelings carefully he will inevitably become guarded, hidden, and emotionally unknown to himself and others and viewed as "cold" and even hostile.

Either way he loses: If he lets it all hang out, he is considered to be immature and to lack self-control. If he contains his emotions he's considered secretive, distant and overly self-controlled.

The Hero-Image Bind

As a growing boy the male will be indoctrinated with the notion of "hero," the epitome of masculine behavior. This entails the willingness on his part to take hazardous risks and to accept challenges to his masculinity even when doing so may result in injury to himself. Behaving "courageously" often means denying instinctive fear and plunging into unnecessarily dangerous situations to prove himself. To validate himself as a male, therefore, he may engage in hazardous, potentially self-destructive behavior. For example, if he is challenged by another male, even if defeat seems certain, and he doesn't accept the challenge, he may accuse himself of cowardice. Coward, in our language, is almost exclusively an adjective applying to men and one that is particularly destructive to the male self-image.

Either way he loses: If he accepts the challenge, assumes the risks, confronts dangers head on, he is very likely eventually to engage in behavior injurious to himself. If he resists or runs away from the challenges he encounters the revulsion and accusation of other young males, particularly peers who will label him "coward," "chicken-shit," "sissy"—accusations that will have a devastating impact on his self-image.

The Companionship Bind

As a boy, the male will be encouraged to play primarily with other boys. He is constantly being urged to participate in and enjoy "masculine" activities, to shun "playing house," playing with dolls, and staying indoors engaging in passive, docile games. He will be a source of great concern and anxiety to his parents if he enjoys, or worse still prefers the company of females. However, as he grows into maturity and becomes an adult male the exact opposite expectation is placed on him. If he prefers or even seems to enjoy too much the companionship of other males he will be considered immature, possibly homosexual. Instead, particularly as a married male he must learn to enjoy "playing house," having his wife as his primary companion and friend. He feels compelled to include her into and make her an integral part of his leisure play activities, which he was conditioned as a boy to enjoy primarily with other boys. These expectations fall within the traditional social definition of a mature male.

Either way he loses: As an adult male, if he behaves in a way that is continuous with his early experiences, he will be seen as immature, rejecting, hostile to women, latently homosexual, or a male chauvinist—particularly if he is married. If he behaves in the way that is expected of him, he will be doing it at the price of denying himself an intrinsic source of pleasure. He often will feel unexpectedly and with no obvious reason resentful, bored, and frustrated. Eventually, he may arrive at a typically male passive-agressive solution. That is, he won't do the things he really wants to do, but he also won't really get into and fully enjoy activities with his woman. Instead, he'll function in a relatively detached, passive manner, sitting at home or elsewhere and doing nothing. He won't please himself, but he won't please his woman either.

The Child-Rearing Bind

If as a father he is heavily involved with his family and tries to take an active part in rearing the children he may clash with his wife over child-rearing philosophy and attitudes. He will be resented for interfering, for not backing up his wife, and for creating dissension. If he lays back, largely staying out of the picture, and tries not to interfere, thereby allowing his wife to be the principle authority in child-rearing, he may be resented for being a passive, uninvolved father and his influence in the family and the depth of his relationship with his children will steadily diminish.

Either way he loses: If he tries to involve himself heavily in the child rearing he may be resented for having a divisive influence. If he tries to stay out of the picture he may be resented for being a passive, uninvolved father.

The Identity Bind

At work, if he is success and achievement-oriented, he will develop a style of being dominant, aggressive, emotionally controlled and detached. At home with his family, however, he will try to be tender, empathic, sensitive, selfless, warm, and caring.

Either way he loses: If he tries to be an emotionally integrated, unified, whole person, he will either be too soft at work or too harsh at home. If he tries to be all things to all people, the aggressor at work and the lover at home, he will have to split up his personality, controlling and monitoring his responses in each setting and paying the price of being overly controlled and only partially himself in both settings.

The Authority Bind

In his work situation, or in the home, if he strives to be democratic, genuinely trying to take into consideration the needs of others and to reconcile the feelings of different people, he may be seen as indecisive and even weak. If he takes on the direct leadership role and behaves in a decisive manner he may be seen as authoritarian and be disliked for this by others.

Either way he loses: If he is sensitive to other people's opinions and needs he inevitably will waver and his decisiveness will suffer. If he assumes responsibility and leadership he may be seen as arbitrary, insensitive to others, and domineering.

The Breadwinner Bind

To be an acceptable husband and father the adult male is taught that he must provide his family with the best life possible. He will be admired and praised for being a good provider and a capable competitor. In the process of striving to make the "good life" a reality, he will be confronted by the complaints of his intimates that he isn't involved enough with them. They will say he always is busy or tired, works too much and, in general, is a neglecting husband and father. He also will be prone to accusing and questioning himself as he succumbs to the compulsive, never-ending routines required for material survival, routines that make involvement with his family increasingly more difficult.

Either way he loses: If he is a hard worker he may be resented by his intimates for being a neglectful family man and for having his values out of place. If he withdraws from the rat race, he will tend to compare himself and may be compared by his family unfavorably with those who are more successful.

The Success Bind

The male is taught to strive for success and achievement and is heavily praised, respected, and admired for being a winner. To accomplish this however, he must be goal-oriented, driven, competitive, and manipulative. Particularly, if he aspires to be a leader or a boss he must learn to be impersonal and detached in his dealings with others. However, he is also taught that to be a good human being he must be warm, open, caring, loving, and sharing. None of these qualities however, are truly compatible with the competitive, success orientation he has also been taught.

Either way he loses: In order to achieve and be successful he must be competitive, which inevitably means alienating himself from others. If he strives to be more human he may learn that all too often, "nice guys finish last!" Therefore, if he chooses to be a success he may end up basically alienated and out of intimate contact with others. If he chooses humanness, he may find himself a failure.

The Career-Ladder Bind

The quest for occupational upward mobility presents another male bind. In order to meet the definition of success he must continue to be upwardly mobile, to strive for promotions and to take on greater and greater responsibility. In the process, however, he often has to give up doing that which he once did best, what originally attracted him to his work, and which gave him the deepest satisfactions. As he advances, he will also find it increasingly more difficult to relate to former co-workers and others who were once his friends. If he contents himself with continuing to do the thing he does best and enjoys most and avoids promotion, he may be seen as unsuccessful and may also make his own future vulnerable to those who will pass him by and who will gain the power positions over him that he neglected to pursue.

Either way he loses: If he maintains upward vocational mobility in the pursuit of success, he may lose the intrinsic satis-factions of doing what he once did best and enjoyed doing most, and may also lose close friends who can no longer comfortably relate to him as a superior. If he allows himself to be passed up by others he may be seen as a failure and may put himself in a potentially vulnerable position.

The Integrity Bind

The man who is honest and direct with others in the work relationship may be criticized for being tactless, undiplomatic, inappropriate, socially naive, and even cruel. If he shapes himself up into the "nice guy," hiding his real feelings behind a smile, a handshake, and a smooth manner, he may be viewed as competent and a good team man but may feel progressively more unreal, phony, and resentful.

Either way he loses: If he is honest, direct and open he stands to jeopardize his job and career. If he plays the "nice guy" and is basically dishonest and manipulative in his responses, he may become successful but he has turned himself into an object and his relationships will become increasingly dehumanized and frustrating.

The Monogamy Bind

As a growing adolescent male and as a young adult, he will be admired and held in esteem by his peers for making many sexual conquests. In the area of sex he'll be oriented to chase, challenge, and conquer. As an adult man married or living in an exclusive relationship with a woman, the chase, challenge, and conquer style will not fit. Instead he will have to live up to the model of the "mature" relationship and he will strive to have a fulfilling, meaningful sexual relationship with one woman, but he may find that he can't fit comfortably into the monogamous model either.

Either way he loses: If he continues in the spirit and direction of chase, challenge, and conquer, he will feel that his relationships are shallow and will be accused of being unable to sustain an intimate relationship. If he keeps himself in the monogamous model he may experience sexual boredom, anxiety over his performance and adequacy, and frustration over not being able to have sex with other women, and may become preoccupied with sexual fantasies.

The Sensuality Bind

As a boy, the male learns that touching, cuddling, stroking, and other expressions of physical affection are primarily for girls and that it is not manly to ask to be kissed, hugged, held, stroked, etc. As an adult male lover however, he learns that sensuality and being a good lover involves the capacity and ability to enjoy freely and comfortably being touched, cuddled, and stroked, and to express physical affection.

Either way he loses: If he is uncomfortable with affectionate contact he may be seen by his partner as a cold, abrupt, harsh, insensitive, and unsensual lover. If he strives to be sensual it may seem forced to his partner and he may not feel naturally comfortable with it himself. He even may begin to become sexually inhibited as he strives to be other than he is. This will impair his performance and he will accuse himself of being an inadequate lover.

The Autonomy Bind

The male is encouraged to be independent and not to lean on others for help. However, he has a deep-rooted need to be nourished and cared for.

Either way he loses: If he resists and refrains from asking for help he will suffer alone in silence, exhausting, and torturing himself fighting uphill battles he can't cope with and draining energies in the process. If he asks for help and allows himself to be dependent he becomes anxious, uncomfortable, and feels vulnerable and therefore feels his masculinity is at stake if he is confused, lost, or troubled.

The Health Bind

As a boy, the male is taught that it is unmasculine to complain about physical symptoms and illness. "Real men" don't give in to their bodily ills and injuries unless the symptoms are severe. Being concerned with health and the body is considered weak, self-indulgent, or hypochondriacal behavior. At the same time he's bombarded with warnings about health and physical fitness.

Either way he loses: If he is sensitive to body distress signals, takes good care of himself, goes to bed readily when fatigued or not feeling well, and refuses to work under those conditions he may be considered hypochondriacal and self-indulgent and his masculinity may be questioned. If he ignores body signals, takes it "like a man," rises above his injuries, and pushes himself until he is forced to stop, he will be considered brave but he may thereby lay the foundations for chronic illness and possibly early death.

The Spontaneity Bind

As an adult the male is often accused of not being spontaneous, of being afraid to let go and be playful and uninhibited. He is told that he is too self-conscious. When he does let go and expresses himself in a spontaneous, uninhibited style he may be likely to make other people uncomfortable and embarrassed.

Either way he loses: If he is serious in his attitude he is told to loosen up, not be so rigid, inhibited, and self-conscious. If he behaves in a spontaneous, free, and uninhibited way, others may become uncomfortable and accuse him of making a fool out of himself, call him childish, and label his behavior inappropriate.

The Priority Bind

If he plays the part of "good guy," who puts the needs of family, friends, and co-workers first he finds that he has little time and energy left for doing the things that please him and are only for his pleasure and benefit. If he puts himself first and emphasizes his own needs and pleasures he will be seen as an uncaring, selfish person.

Either way he loses: If he gives priority to the needs of others and puts himself second, he will indeed have little time for his own pleasures and self-development, and may feel like a martyr. If he puts himself first he will be seen as selfish and may begin to feel guilty.

The Growth Bind

The aware adult male has a need to grow, change and expand. On the other hand, he has a strong need for security and has a responsibility to those who depend on him.

Either way he loses: If he allows himself to grow by changing careers, forming new relationships, or altering his lifestyle, he jeopardizes his security and risks destroying his relationships, and may be seen by others and himself as irresponsible. If he denies his growth impulses, he feels trapped, stagnant and may be chided by his intimates and called boring and set in his ways.

The binds that ensnare the male, who will then also tend to ensnare the female, are a fact of his existence. The first step in coping with this phenomenon is open recognition and acknowledgement of these binds. For most males, consciousness of these contradictions and conflicts tends to be blocked out and repressed for self-protection. However, there is an inevitable price to be paid for this, either in a sudden eruption and falling apart of one's life under the weight of these gathering frustrations, or consciousness may never occur and the destructive impact will manifest itself through physiological or psychological symptoms. Deterioration will be caused by the impact of these constant hidden stresses—stresses that slowly wear away at him. In every conflict there is a real need or impulse that underlies the bind. Release from impossible binds can occur if the male reclaims the deepest needs, feelings, or impulses that lie behind his defenses—recognizing them, accepting them as being a part of himself, albeit a threatening part, and then consciously deciding to what extent he is willing or can risk being true to the real self lying behind the defense.

Undoubtedly, the re-owning of the real self will precipitate a crisis in the lives of all men who have allowed themselves to be bound up in these annihilating conflicts. It may therefore be necessary to acknowledge the need for help with these struggles and to seek it from a competent psychotherapist. At this stage in our culture the price of awareness seems to be far smaller than the incredibily high price that the male is paying for the dubious bliss of unconsciousness.

7. The Destruction
Of The Male Body

The microbe is nothing, the terrain is everything.[1]
—Louis Pasteur

There are, I believe, three basic processes that contribute to the physical deterioration of the male body. They are intellectualization, macho rigidity, and guilt.

Intellectualization

By intellectualization I mean the kind of orientation to one's body and health that in effect says, "I will accept it as true only if you can prove it to me objectively with scientific data or if it is spoken by an authority in the field." I have no objection to the scientific approach per se; I would not like to live in a society of witch doctors and healing charlatans. However, I am equally stunned that, for example, it requires a ten-year study by the Surgeon General and millions of dollars in research money to prove that cigarette smoking may be hazardous to your health. And even after the findings came out controversy about its validity continues. While I am aware that smoking undoubtedly affects people differently and I myself have no strong positive or negative feelings about smoking, I ask myself, "Doesn't the man who smokes know how it is affecting him and whether or not it is impairing his health? Is he getting no warning signals or messages of discomfort from his body?" In other words, it seems clear that we have become so alienated from our bodies that we believe that only an objective, "scientific," totally intellectualized approach can tell us how a particular substance affects us.

By intellectualization I also mean that state of affairs that causes us to be so out of touch with our bodies that we constantly must consult an authority figure in order to know what to do with them. We look to a physician to order us to bed when we are ill and to tell us when we can get out of bed and resume our everyday existences; to tell us what kinds of foods to eat and in what quantity; how much and what kind of exercise to take, etc, etc. This same phenomenon can produce a situation where a man may "feel great" one day and suffer a heart attack the next. I always wonder when I hear of such instances, where were the body's messages of distress all during the time it was weakening to the point of this total collapse?

A vivid example of this phenomenon has remained in my mind from my years as a graduate student. I remember reading a study in a child development textbook on the self-selection of diets by infants. The study was conducted with a group of children who had just been weaned. It followed these children for six years. Many of them, when the study began, had rickets, and were underweight and poorly nourished. In her study, researcher Clara M. Davis had a wide variety of natural foods set in front of the children three times a day. These included, among others: orange juice, peaches, carrots, beef, fish, oatmeal, milk, bananas, and sea salt. No canned or incomplete foods were used. Cooking was done without the loss of soluble nutritional substances and without the addition of salt or seasonings. Combinations of food such as soups or bread were not used, to insure that whatever food was eaten was chosen for itself alone.

Food was never offered to the infant directly or even by suggestion. When and only when the infant reached for it or pointed to it was it spooned up and fed to him by a nurse and only if the baby opened his mouth freely. The child could eat as he liked, with fingers or with a spoon and no comments were made about his manners. The children ate what and how they liked and in the quantity they wished. The combinations they chose often were strange by traditional standards. Breakfast might have been orange juice and liver. Supper might have been bananas and eggs. But all of the children thrived, regardless of the "crazy" combinations. Constipation was unknown. Over the six-year period there were no serious illnesses among any of the children. All of the infants with rickets were cured. After an initial exploratory phase of tasting different foods, the children chose by "instinct" those foods whose caloric and vitamin intake and acid-alkaline balance was apparently superb. A roentgenologist at the Children's Memorial Hospital wrote to researcher Davis that, "The beautifully calcified bones in roentgenograms of your young children stand out so well that I have no trouble picking them out when seen at a distance."[2] Another doctor, in a published article in the *Journal of Pediatrics* stated, "I saw them on a number of occasions and they were the finest group of specimens from the physical and behavior standpoint that I have ever seen in children of that age."[3]

This study, conducted in the thirties, was criticized because it only included natural foods. Rather than taking note of its incredible results and following through on the implications one critic suggested that there would be no way of knowing whether there was such a thing as "natural body wisdom" unless the children were allowed to roam freely in an environment that also offered processed foods such as popsicles, soft drinks, cookies, macaroni, etc.[4] The heavy import of the study was ignored: the body will choose what it needs naturally, if body chemistry is not subverted by the use of processed and other "artificial" foods. The study had not, in this case, apparently fulfilled the "logic" of science. Consequently, it has become largely forgotten and ignored.

We insist that all our insights and learning come through the magic of science, via the "magic" pill or the "magic" surgical technique. The fantasy is that we will be saved by the brilliance of a researcher, holed up in a cubicle who, after years of travail, will have the "eureka" experience, announcing to the world that he has found the "fountain of youth and health" in some chemical compound. We accept that fantasy. However, it seems increasingly clear that: 1) The responsibility for health and long life is one's own; 2) No authority has better answers than one's own body; 3) If we get sick we laid the foundation for it; and 4) We had better explore our physical habits, emotional repressions, environment, and interpersonal relationships for answers to health. We are hooked on the magic of science and vigorously resist seeing ourselves in the daily process of creating our own illnesses and our own death. Even many of the most brilliant of men seem totally blocked and blinded to seeing that they are the daily creators of their bodily states.

In a sense, we still live with an antiquated consciousness that perceives disease and illness as an entity in itself, divorced from all that came before it except the mysterious, invisible virus or germ that has attacked us. The prevailing belief still seems to be that disease just suddenly appears and we are the pathetic, random victims of some capricious force in nature, populated by a nest of invisible enemies. I personally resist that picture of my environment that says that danger to my body lurks everywhere—on unwashed fruit, on the floor, in the air, in other people's breath. Rather, it is my belief that an individual, in rhythm with his body and its needs, will thrive, and that "the terrain is everything," meaning the ability to listen to, respect, and respond to the demands of the body.

It also appears to me that the contemporary male has over-identified with the machines he has created and approaches his body as if it were one of his mechanical creations. He treats his body as if it were made up of a series of disconnected component parts which, like his automobile, have to be treated or "repaired" separately. This is yet another manifestation of the phenomenon of intellectualization. That is, you "cure" an automobile by "treating" or replacing its separate, malfunctioning parts; the battery, the alternator, the head gasket, etc. This is also the way the typical male approaches his ailing body. He sees no connection between one ailment and the other; between the state of his gums, the condition of his stomach, the condition of his eyes and the condition of his liver. Each, in his mind, is an entity to be treated separately. His body is not seen as a unity. It is as if each part of the body had its own blood supply, its own chemical environment. There is no awareness that in reality, there only may be varying *degrees* of health and that when the body is in a deteriorated condition all parts will be effected even though one part may bear the diagnostic label because it is the weakest, most vulnerable link and has been affected the most.

Another manifestation of intellectualization is the tendency to cling to authority figures. I believe this is in part the result of the tremendously contradictory information given to people. It has probably increased their confusion, helplessness, and vulnerability. This is much like the child who regresses and becomes disoriented, withdrawn, and dependent because he cannot structure his environment in the face of the contradictory reactions he gets from his parents. One day he is pun-

ished for doing the same thing he was praised for doing the
day before; or one day he is told something he does is good
and the next day told that the same thing is bad.

In like fashion, the public has been bombarded with contradictory research findings. One day they are informed that
meat proteins are the building blocks of life and then they are
told that meat may be a factor in causing cancer or high cholesterol. The virtues of vitamin supplements are hailed by
some, while others tell us that they may be poisonous. The
sun is described one time as a healing, protective influence
and as a producer of skin cancer the next. Some researchers
tell us food additives are poisonous, others say that they are
harmless. Extensive post-operative bed rest is recommended
by some and pooh-poohed by others. Some say milk belongs
in every body while others tell us milk is harmful for adults.
Etc. Etc.

The process of intellectualization, which affects the way
most men approach their bodies, is therefore a major factor in
its destruction. To view one's body as a thing, a piece of
machinery, rather than seeing one's well-being and ills as part
of the total process of one's life, is to ignore the way in which
human beings *create* whatever state of health they are in.

Macho Rigidity

The destruction of the male body as a result of macho rigidity
manifests itself in countless ways. Though men die from almost every major disease at a significantly higher rate than
women, study after study indicates that women complain of
significantly more symptoms and go to doctors more often. In
effect, what this says is that men are significantly more out of
touch with the body's warning signals. As one study pointed
out about women: "A greater number of minor complaints
could be attributed purely to greater awareness of, or concern
with, physical symptoms."[5]

One study on the psychosomatic aspects of symptom patterns among surgery patients revealed that women respond to
stress before surgery by acting out their emotions in clear behaviors of expressed fear, anger, or depression. Men, on the

other hand, tended to keep a stiff upper lip, and consequently
had, in general, higher levels of anxiety.[6]

Despite the fact that men, almost from birth on, seem to
react more sensitively to stress than women,[7] one researcher
discovered that women can perceive the signs of stress significantly more often than men. He had 617 families report on
the reactions to stress that they perceived in themselves. These
reactions included, "face feels hot or flushed," "nervous stomach," "sweating palms," "lumps in throat or dryness in
mouth," "cold hands and/or feet," "general restlessness,"
"general body sweating," "increased heart rate," "frequent uri-
nation," and "awareness of heartbeat." Of these ten stress
signs men experienced only "sweating palms" more often
than women. The women however, reported "flushed face,"
"nervous stomach," "cold hands and/or feet," "frequent urina-
tion," and "awareness of heartbeat," significantly more often
than men.[8] These findings suggest that men tend to block out
the signs of stress, while women are more aware of them.

All of these findings say that men are quite out of touch
with their bodies. Consequently, they have almost every major
disease leading to death at a much higher rate than women.
They have a tendency to be "suddenly" struck by a major
illness such as a heart attack. They block out the symptoms of
malaise until the illness is so overwhelming that it disables
them completely.

This situation is partially the outgrowth of early conditioning that teaches boys that it is "sissy behavior" to complain of
body pains and also encourages him to deny and resist the fact
of illness and injuries as long as possible. One cultural definition of being a "real boy" or a hero is that he carries on,
whether in a football game, a fight, or in his activities *in spite*
of his injuries and symptoms. This is the subtle and unconscious condition of the male in our culture. He is taught very
early in life that it is unmanly to be ill, unmanly to complain,
and unmanly to ask for help.

A story about Rudolph Valentino, published at the time of
his death, points up in a poignant though revealing fashion the
macho orientation and how it remains a part of the male until
the day of his death.

Valentino, as a silent screen star, was the very personifica-
tion of the macho male hero and stud. He had collapsed suddenly in his apartment and several hours later underwent op-

erations for a gastric ulcer and appendicitis. When he became conscious, it was reported that his first words were a question about his courage. He felt it had been impugned in an editorial in the *Chicago Tribune* titled, "Pink Powder Puffs." The editorial had prompted Valentino to challenge the anonymous writer to a duel, however, nothing ever came of the challenge.

Shortly before Valentino died, as he came out of the anesthetic, it was reported that he looked up at his doctor and asked, "Doctor, am I a 'Pink Powder Puff'?" The doctor replied, "No, indeed, you have been very brave."⁹

I have often noticed families where the mother constantly complains of her symptoms and her illnesses and goes to the doctor frequently, often acting as if she were on the verge of death. Her "strong" and "silent" husband, however, would rarely if ever be heard complaining of his ills; if he did everyone would know it was serious. He just carries on, manfully priding himself on not giving in to his body's distress signals. He also gets seriously ill or dies in his fifties while his complaining wife is still going strong in her seventies.

There are other reasons for the male tendency to deny and resist his body's signals of distress. His dread of passivity, which he unconsciously associates with femininity and homosexuality, is critical. It leads to a reluctance and resistance to going to bed and staying there when he is not feeling well. Instead he delays it until he is literally knocked off his feet and forced to lie down. His badge of honor is that he never misses a day of work, so he ignores the distress signals in order to keep on achieving and competing. He's proving that he's a man and can resist, ignore, and overcome signs of illness.

A cultural archetype and contemporary illustration of this phenomenon is the super macho professional athlete, like the football player. Pain-killing drugs are regularly administered to the injured victims of this violent body contact sport and the player is immediately thrown back in the game. Upon return he is greeted by the appreciative roar of the crowd that seems to be saying in unison, "What a man!"

Even many of the non-injured players in the super macho sports such as wrestling, football, and weight-lifting are widely known for whipping their tired bodies into play by taking amphetamines ("speed") to get them going and barbiturates to help bring them back down. In between, they take anabolic steroids to build up their muscles. These steroids reportedly have side effects such as testicular atrophy, liver damage, and edema.[10]

All these illustrations directly relate to the macho pressure to continue to perform at all costs and to ignore or deny body pain. In the macho mind a day in bed sick means:

1) His territory is threatened and someone might usurp his position.

2) Someone might discover he really isn't needed or might try to replace him.

3) Each day in bed is money lost.

4) He's not a capable warrior and doesn't hold up under pressure.

The male resistance to being sick also ties in with his fear of dependency, particularly on women. This makes illness a kind of shameful, embarrassing experience, particularly for the married male. While he may allow his wife to cater to him for a short while, his anxiety mounts as he hears echoes that warn him not to be tied to mother's apron strings or act like a helpless baby.

While sick in bed, the married male may also sense the conscious or unconscious resentment of his wife. In the traditional marriage dynamic, the woman sometimes fantasizes her husband as a superman, protector, and provider. Seeing him prone and ill in bed may be subliminally threatening and traumatizing to her. It can shatter her illusion and need to see him as omnipotent. The unconscious message of discomfort he may receive from her may add to his own guilt and discomfort about being sick and motivate him to get out of bed as quickly as possible.

While it is perfectly acceptable for the woman in our culture to preen and admire herself in front of a mirror and to spend considerable time caring for her body with long baths, stretching exercises, the use of body creams, etc., the male generally feels uncomfortable and embarrassed about giving his body extensive tender loving care. Again, it is not in line with his masculine self-image. A female who so indulged herself would be considered to be behaving in an appropriate manner. The male however, would be suspect, accused of being narcissistic or worse still a latent homosexual. This accusation often has been hurled at weight-lifters by those upset at seeing them indulge themselves at great lengths in front of a mirror.

A recent study on male and female body image pointed out that women have ". . . a more clearly differentiated body concept. . . . ," that they tend to value their bodies more than men do and tend to show more approval of themselves in front of full-length mirrors. The over-all finding was that women clearly had a "higher evaluation of their bodies."[11]

Even diet is heavily colored by sex-role or gender expectations. There are certain foods which are considered "masculine," such as steak. Many men react negatively to eating "health foods" or light vegetarian diets. These diets are often referred to disdainfully by macho males as "rabbit food." This rigidity in the realm of diet is both paradoxical and tragic. It is paradoxical because many men, particularly white-collar workers, continue to eat as if they were the hunter-warriors of old, and, in the process, rapidly destroy their bodies.

The association between heavy meat-eating and masculinity may prove to be unfortunate in many ways. It was recently reported to the American Cancer Society that cancer related to nutrition accounts for 30 per cent of cancer in men. This report cited the habit of eating red meat as a major factor.[12] Cancer of the bowel, which is the most common form of cancer, has also been linked to the eating of beef, a food which is known to contribute to high cholesterol.[13]

A recent report by a physician from the Mayo Clinic on the "longevity diet" of the future was presented at an A.M.A. conference on the medical aspects of sports. It outlined the destructiveness of the macho orientation toward food. Specifically, among the important conclusions were the following:

High protein diets shorten life.

Vitamin supplements can be poisonous.

Muscle proteins *cannot* be increased by eating more meat, drinking milk shakes with eggs, or by eating other high protein foods.

The "longevity diet" of the future will have little or no new ingredients added, but much of what is commonly eaten today will be omitted.

It also debunked the famous male myth that eating meat gives strength. "The fact is meat is not strength," the report said. Eating high protein foods and swallowing extra vitamins, rather than being helpful are harmful to the body. The false reasoning of the macho athlete goes something like this: "Meat is muscle, a person is what he eats, and therefore, he will increase his muscle mass and strength if he eats meat." The report concluded that the saddest part of all this is that once these habits have been learned, the chances of unlearning them is very slim.[14]

Women seem to be much more flexible and less self-destructive in the matters of diet. While they can justifiably eat a heavier diet than their white-collar husbands if they are active doing the physical labor involved in caring for children and maintaining a home, they tend to eat much less and are also less resistant to a diet centered around salads and other light foods.

At a health spa I go to in Mexico that serves only vege-tarian food I have often noted the pained and deprived faces of many men who are reacting negatively to eating vegetables. In the evening they eagerly go to town to eat lobster and steak and to drink beer or liquor—real "male" food.

The "real man" pats his mid-region and prides himself on having an "iron stomach." That means he believes he can put any garbage into it and it won't affect him. This belief is short-sighted macho ignorance and rigidity.

Perhaps because of their great anxiety about intimacy or closeness with other males, or the fear of transparency, men seem to require liquor in order to relax when socializing with associates. They meet at bars or in a restaurant over a drink and then proceed to drink continuously while they are to-gether. When they eat, they eat "macho style," chops, ribs, or some other rich "masculine" food. Women however, seem to be able to socialize comfortably and casually for hours with each other over a cup of coffee or tea. Their anxiety over intimacy and transparency is not nearly as great and feelings do not need to be numbed in order to make the interaction comfortable.

The male competing in the working world and trying to get ahead and carve out his piece of territory must also learn to heavily control his emotions, play the role of "nice guy," and experience the emotional stress of constantly having to make decisions. He pays a heavy price for this "privilege" on a psy-chosomatic level.

The "glories" of being an executive were researched in a

study conducted with monkeys. Two monkeys were placed in restraining chairs with one monkey being assigned the role of executive. The "executive" monkey was given a lever which he learned to press in order to prevent shocks being administered to both himself and the other monkey. After twenty-three days of a continuous six hours on-six hours off schedule the "executive" monkey suddenly died. An autopsy revealed an ulcer—a large perforation in the wall of the duodenum, the upper part of the small intestine near its junction with the stomach. The monkey in the other restraining chair, who was not making decisions, was not affected.[15]

A recent study of psychosomatic illness concluded, many events precursing illnesses are ". . . part and parcel of American values—achievement, success, materialism, and self-reliance."[16] All this macho rigidity in the realm of emotions is by definition also part and parcel of being an American male. The price paid is incredibly high.

An exploration of the personality characteristics that are associated with males who get cancer (male rate is 40 per cent higher over-all than the female and considerably greater for specific sites such as the lungs) is particularly instructive in terms of understanding the impact of the masculine ethos on the body. One study of the personalities of males who were victims of lung cancer found that these patients "have a poor outlet for emotional discharge and that they tend to conceal or bottle up their emotional difficulties."[17]

Emotional denial, that causes the male cancer patient to delay seeking help, has also been consistently noted. It was discovered that cancer victims tended to deny anything that could be construed as embarrassing or socially undesirable, such as that:

1) Their feelings were hurt easier than most people's.
2) They often got sick to their stomach.
3) They had upsetting nightmares.
4) They felt alone in the world.
5) No one really understood them.
6) Their wives were not satisfied with their accomplishments in life.[18]

Another illustration is the typical personality pattern of the person who develops hypertension. It is one that could apply to a vast number of men and might account for the high incidence of male heart attacks. Clinical data suggests that hypertensives are caught in painful conflicts with no consistent outlet for expression of their feelings available to them. That is, while they are deeply resentful underneath, these feelings come through only occasionally in a burst of rage. Otherwise, they have no regular way of expressing their aggressive tendencies.[19] Indeed, in the "nice guy" world of business there is no acceptable way. This conflict characterizes the lives of many men, at work as well as at home.

Other studies on male patients with coronary artery disease have found them to be persons with excessively competitive and persistent needs for recognition.

The price of macho rigidity—including the resistance to asking for help, the fear of dependency, the resistance against passivity, notions about what constitutes "masculine" foods, reluctance to pamper oneself and the bottling up of emotions—is high indeed in terms of the damage done to the body. To alter these patterns, the male will have to look to himself and summon his own desire to survive and enjoy his life. He cannot, as some well-intentioned doctors have suggested, rely on his wife to help him to overcome these macho patterns. Though the traditional wife may consciously seek to be helpful in many ways, she may also be an integral part of the problem. That is, while her conscious intentions may be helpful, she may have a significant investment in her husband's worldly success and in his playing out the role of "macho-superman." The drive for health, self-care, and longevity must therefore emerge as a purely selfish one on the male's part. He must do it because he delights in the good feelings in his body when he treats himself well and he must make that a primary motivation in his life.

I recently came across a study done with rats entitled, "Voodoo Death: Some New Thoughts on an Old Phenomenon."[20] This study that explored the phenomenon of "sudden death" from "unknown causes" provides a particularly apt analogy. Sudden death without any prior clear inpending signs seems to afflict men in our culture all too frequently.

In this study, in which rats were restrained and put in a stress situation which allowed no opportunities for escape, no flight or fight possibilities, making the situation a hopeless one, the rats began to behave as if they'd literally given up.

Such, I believe, may be the inner state of many men in our culture when they suddenly and seemingly inexplicably drop dead. Their death is their final expression of hopelessness, of being stuck with no way out, and of finally having given in and given up. Whether the hopelessness sets in during his "success" voyage when he encapsulates himself so much that emotional nourishment from others and emotional expression from himself becomes totally blocked, or whether it sets in after he has been sent out to pasture, fired or retired when all he ever knew was how to work, sudden death is the mark of the male in our culture, suffocating in the rigid binds of his macho pose.

I fully concur with a feminist and free-lance writer who recently wrote: "I don't want to wear a handsome suit, carry a briefcase, and anticipate clogged arteries at age 40."[21]

Guilt

It is not ususual for a man, after a year or so of marriage, to pat his stomach and to point jokingly and pridefully to the weight he has gained, while describing what a good cook his wife is. What he is *really* saying is, "Look how well she feeds me. That *proves* she loves me."

It is my observation that the typical "macho" male and his "earth mother" wife often have really very little in common. However, both have accepted the traditional definitions of "mature" and "meaningful" relationships and frequently are trying valiantly to live up to the image that they carry inside themselves—that of "sharing" and "doing together." What can happen as a result is that they have to force it because it doesn't come naturally. They end up relating to each other in regressive ways, the most common pattern being that of mother (the wife) and well-fed child (the husband).

Since he is usually physically stronger and more athletic and since she is typically not openly aggressive and may not want to "damage" his ego by being overtly competitive with him, there is not much deep or lasting pleasure in sharing physically competitive pursuits. In fact, any kind of male-female directly competitive interaction tends to be verboten and anxiety-producing for both. "Macho" males are taught to treat their women softly and tenderly. So perhaps they go through a phase early in their marriage of hiking, playing tennis, and going on skiing trips. But invariably they give this up or begin to do it less and less.

Though they may make a pact at the beginning of the relationship that each will have free time on their own to see friends and engage in separate activities, after some of these bursts into freedom the male often retreats from independent activity out of guilt and also perhaps because of the resentful vibrations he may get from his wife. He therefore gives up his "extracurricular" activities with his associates or friends. In part, this is also because he feels guilty when he is having a good time and not sharing his experience with his wife, as he tells himself a "good" husband should.

In order therefore to find things that the two of them can share and enjoy comfortably, he begins to engage in primarily the more passive activities such as eating out, going to the theatre, movies, or museums, taking long walks, picnicking, watching television, visiting friends, or having friends over for dinner—and increasingly neglects the more active ones he may have engaged in as a single male. For the married couple, when friends come over it becomes an endless round of eating, drinking, smoking, talking, and sitting. After a few hours everyone's feeling lethargic and inert and the evening ends.

Consequently, after about the first five to ten years of marriage, I have noted that many males become caricatures of their former physical selves. They are paunchy, slowed down, balding, and with an assortment of physical complaints such as backaches and fatigue.

In general, liberation of the male consciousness is partially predicated on the liberation of the male body. A man whose physical awareness is inhibited by guilt, who relies on his wife to "take care of him," who is out of touch with, distrustful and unmindful of his body's signals, who intellectualizes rather than responds to his body's messages, who represses his emotions and pays the price in terms of psychosomatic illnesses, and who maintains rigid macho habit patterns in relation to both males and females is on a path of self-destruction.

How To Respect Your Body

1. Learn to listen to, trust, and respond to your body's messages. Do not numb, disguise, hide, or deny them. They are your survival signals and the price of ignoring them may be chronic, irreversible damage to your body.
2. Learn to relish the joys of healthy passivity, napping when you're tired, going to bed when you're fatigued or not feeling well, and delighting in the joys of sleeping. This is not unmale or a waste of time. Do not stimulate a worn-out body by kicking it back into motion the way you might a tired horse.
3. Learn to separate masculinity from the eating of certain foods. You can be just as much of a man with a salad as with a steak.
4. Release yourself from the notion that says feeding you means she loves you. Get your love directly. She can love you and you can love her without proving it through food stuffing.
5. Break your macho-oriented interaction patterns with other males. Learn to relate and communicate with them openly and playfully rather than behind a shot of alcohol and a cigarette.
6. Learn to prepare your own foods, according to your needs. Your wife or girl friend is not your mother and you are not a helpless child. Eat what you need, when you need it.
7. Spend some time each day caring for your body and looking at yourself in the mirror. React with alarm at signs that you are not taking care of yourself and praise yourself for looking good, feeling supple and healthy. When your body deteriorates you deteriorate because *you are your body*.
8. Refuse to sit passively in the evening watching television and munching on goodies, if that bores you. Be active if you feel energetic, go to sleep if you're tired. If you're married or living with a woman, don't just sit there thinking you are accommodating her by being passive under

the illusion that it constitutes involvement and means that you are being a good lover, husband, or father.

9. Take all the time alone that you require for going to the gym, playing outdoors or at the beach, evenings or weekends.

10. Learn to say "no" to activities and social events you don't enjoy but are engaging in to be "nice." Avoid cocktail parties or long dinner parties and sitting around in people's living rooms unless you truly enjoy the experience.

11. Find a person who is older and in top physical health, even if your impulse is to dismiss him as a kook or a fanatic, and learn from him. Ask him how he does it and keep yourself open to the possibility that he may know something that you don't know.

12. Learn to be selfish about your body. One ultimate value of life will always be health. A vibrantly healthy man is an attractive man. Without it joylessness and meaninglessness become an increasingly present reality.

8. The Success Trip:
A Fantasy Portrait

> "What are faces?
> You don't build an empire by remembering faces!"[1]
> —Big Daddy
> —*Cat on a Hot Tin Roof*

A young boy learns to value himself in terms of achievements, sucesses, and victories. The message is brought home to him constantly, both in direct and indirect ways: When he runs faster, speaks better, wins a game, reads earlier, gets a higher grade, shows more strength, or does anything that demonstrates his superiority over other young boys, his father proudly calls him "my son" and together with his mother they brag about his accomplishments to others.

Periodically, however, he'll be reminded that even though he does certain things well he must never rest on his laurels, because he lives in a world that only has room for the best, a world with little space or sympathy for a loser. A loser is defined by the saying, "A miss is as good as a mile." In effect, anyone who isn't a winner is a loser.

Indirectly, he will get the same kinds of messages when he hears his mother talking about how good someone else's boy is at doing something. He'll come to understand the underlying message there which is, "Wouldn't it be great if you were that good too!"

Throughout those early years when he does win or succeed he will be praised and otherwise rewarded. He will be treated in a special way that makes him feel proud of himself and good inside.

However, when he loses, fails, acts in a clumsy or ineffectual, weak, or incompetent way, he'll feel particularly his father's, and often also his mother's, disapproval and rejection.

Perhaps this won't be expressed directly. He may be responded to in a solicitous tone in which the rejection is hidden behind "supportive" words such as, "It's O.K. You'll do better next time," "Nobody can win them all," "It's not whether you win or lose, its how you play the game." The rejection however is clearly implied in subtle tones by the fact that when he does win or succeed he is responded to with enthusiasm. When he doesn't, even though the words are "kind," the emotional tone behind them is muted, lukewarm, or negative.

If his parents are not psychologically sophisticated, the feedback he will receive when he doesn't perform well will be more direct. Perhaps he will be rejected in favor of a better performing sibling. Or, he'll be put down with derogatory comments about his intelligence or adequacy.

As a growing boy he will increasingly internalize parental and other attitudes that he hears until he becomes his own parent. That is, he will develop his own inner voice that will say nice things to him that make him feel good when he performs well or wins, and will insult, gnaw at him, and put him down when he doesn't do as well or better than his peers.

He is now in the process of building a permanent, latent reservoir of self-hate and abuse that threatens to pour through whenever he fails to achieve. This reservoir will dampen even his greatest triumphs, as even in "victory" he will always be focusing on those who are "better" than himself. He now has a built-in motor that will forever be driving him toward success goals.

His moods and emotions will become intertwined with his successes and failures. When he has won, proven himself, or performed well he'll feel elated. When he fails or disappoints he will feel depressed, ashamed, and embarrassed.

In time however, he will learn to control and hide all of his feelings until his spontaneous or genuine responses are replaced by appropriately controlled ones. The ones that "work," make him seem strong and enable him to project the appropriate image.

At first these emotional controls will be erratic. Periodically, feelings will break through that he fears have spoiled his image as a "winner." Increasingly however, these will get sorted out until the un-self-conscious moments become fewer and fewer while he becomes more and more polished. This process of becoming polished will feel so good to him that he won't even be aware of how he is totally losing touch with himself, giving up his true responses for the well-programmed ones designed to make him a better success machine.

Even his closest friendships with other boys will be contaminated by the fact that he's constantly being compared to them by others and he is constantly comparing himself to them. Being friends feels good but being better becomes even more important.

As he grows older, other boys are seen less as friends and more as competitors, potential threats to his own success pursuits. Therefore, he begins to become more guarded around them, hiding his weaknesses, inadequacies, and vulnerabilities. When his friends become too emotional, he becomes uncomfortable. He won't feel he can trust a friend who can't control his emotions.

As he becomes a young adult, finishes school, and goes out into the "real" world, he finds that people are attractive to him, perhaps without even his conscious awareness, in terms of how they enhance his image as a successful man. He'll be attracted to the girl he feels will make him look good and he'll want to be seen with and accepted by the most successful and popular men.

It's time to "grow up" and get married. Where his attraction to women used to be based primarily on the physical, for a marriage partner he chooses a more "sensible," stable, reliable, attractive woman whom he feels proud to introduce to his parents and friends.

While sex always seemed to be so important, other things will now seem to be even more important. He chooses a woman he can count on, who seems to have a relaxed, comforting personality, one who will be an asset to him on his success journey.

He marries her and she "stabilizes" him. His energies now are being channeled into his success trip. He's ready for the climb. By now, he's become a fairly well-oiled machine. His public responses are smooth and socially appropriate. Only his wife gets an occasional glimpse of his uncontrolled parts, when he rages over some small incident, pouts like a child, or becomes cold and withdrawn.

Some years into his success trip, he senses himself becoming increasingly predictable and repetitive in the things he does and says. While the climb upward keeps him on his toes, excited and anxious, his relationship to his wife, his friends, and himself is beginning to feel stagnant and somewhat boring. However, he accepts that as part of the reality of becoming a "mature" adult. Though it bothers him occasionally in moments of restlessness and boredom, it doesn't bother him enough to risk giving up anything in order to change.

When he's not working he's with his family or socializing as a married couple. There isn't enough time for having his own intimate friends, male or female. That kind of need even seems childish and unnecessary to him. His whole life is fast becoming his work and his family.

By now his relationship with most males is distant and guarded. He's even a little paranoid about most of them. Not a "crazy" paranoid but a "reality"-oriented one. That is, as he climbs the success ladder, he finds himself looking behind to see who is moving up on him. He'll be watching those on his level to see if they're moving ahead faster than he or blocking his forward progress. And he'll be looking at those above cautiously and insecurely, for they have power over him and can affect his future. He's worried about what they think of him and whether or not they disapprove of what he's doing.

Looking behind, at the side, and above will create in him a chronic tension and anxiety, a sense of guardedness and jeopardy that will make it difficult, if not impossible, to have a close, trusting relationship with most other men.

The situation with his family is beginning to show strain. His wife is complaining because he doesn't spend enough time at home and that even when he's around he seems to be preoccupied and tends to ignore her.

He hears her complaints and they put him into conflict. When he's working hard to succeed, he's feeling guilty about depriving his family. When he tries to let go and relax more at home he gets anxious feelings about work that prevent him from really enjoying himself. The conflict makes him feel resentful and a little bit desperate.

While he hears his wife complaining that he spends too little time with the family, he can justify the increasing amount of time he spends at work with the knowledge that if the money did stop coming in she'd really have something to complain about.

At work things are beginning to move very well—financially and status-wise. However, it's not as satisfying and fulfilling as he imagined it would be to have more money and position. It doesn't even make him feel very secure.

Quite the opposite. Much of his energy and concerns are now going toward trying to hold on to what he's got. Even though he has more than he ever had before, including a home, an expensive car, investments and money in the bank he feels more insecure than ever about losing his standard of living. The prospect of going backward and doing without what he now has is terrifying to him.

When he's at home he's withdrawn, detached, and passive—in stark contrast to the assertive way the outside world sees him. He blames it on fatigue and overwork.

His wife is pressuring him to open up more, to tell her what he's thinking and feeling, because his quietness troubles her. This puts him into constant conflict that makes him rage inside when she starts to push him to get involved. He doesn't feel like talking, and forcing himself into it is painful.

Besides, if he told her some of the things he was thinking, particularly his fantasies about other women, she couldn't handle it anyway. The safest way to go, he decides, is to just be around enough so that she knows he's trying and fill her in on as much as he comfortably can to keep her happy. He hates himself for being so closed and manipulative but he can't see any other way that feels safe.

He is well into his success trip by now and rather than success softening him toward others it's toughened him and made him more cynical. He used to tell himself that once he got secure, he'd start to be more honest and real with people, maybe even reclaim some of the idealism he felt as an adolescent. But now, he's too busy holding on to what he's got and he's afraid he might peril everything he built up if he created "bad" vibes. Besides, it no longer feels like it's worth the hassle and he doesn't really care enough to risk much. He tells himself that he and his family come first and are the major reason why he continues. He's not about to threaten everything that he's worked so hard for.

Those idealistic and romantic feelings he once had about life are now buried behind an "objective" view of reality. Instead of becoming more liberal as he starts to "make it," he surprises himself by becoming more conservative, both politically and in his attitude toward crime, hedonistic living, etc.

His "objective" eye on the world had caused him to see it increasingly in the way that his father saw it. "It's a dog eat dog world." "Only the strong survive." "Nice guys finish last." "Every man for himself."

All of the rough edges are gone from his worldly face. He's playing everything close to the chest and has become totally guarded about what goes on inside himself. He doesn't reveal his fears, frustrations, and anxieties to anyone, because he feels it would only be a waste and others wouldn't understand or know how to handle it. Besides, it would be "out of character" for him.

Even those he calls friends couldn't say that they really know him. They like him and think of him as a pleasant, "nice guy," but he knows that they don't see his real self—the driving, sometimes ruthless, sometimes frightened, sometimes lonely, sometimes horny man. All they see is the tip of the iceberg. If anybody asked his friends to try and define him, they'd probably wind up admitting that he's pretty much unknown to them as a person.

He rationalizes his loneliness and isolation by telling himself that he's basically a "private" person. He's not very fond of most of the people he knows anyway. They seem phony and preoccupied with themselves, so what's the point of letting any of them get close.

One major irony of the success trip for him is that while he wants to be promoted and to move up the ladder he's discovering a painful truth. The higher he goes in status, the less competent he feels at what he's doing, and the more worried he is that he won't be able to perform to standard.

It bothers him particularly because he recognizes that "proving himself" is a never-ending game that gets harder to play, not easier. He can never prove enough and instead of feeling good about past accomplishments his major concerns are always tied up with whether he'll be able to meet the new, more difficult challenge.

The vague, chronic, underlying feelings of anxiety are becoming stronger. Consequently, it's becoming more difficult for him to make decisions. His memory is getting poorer and if he doesn't write things down he feels he wouldn't remember a thing. This makes him feel less secure about himself. Maybe he's getting prematurely old, he thinks.

He's worried that those who work with him will begin to see through him. He already has grave doubts about whether they respect him. In his fantasies, he imagines that they see him as a phony and a manipulator, because that's how he often sees himself. And then there's that gnawing fear that one day he'll do something—he doesn't know what—and in one fell swoop he'll blow everything he's spent years building up.

A few years ago he started having a drink or two at lunchtime, mainly at business lunches. Now he finds himself drinking every day at lunch and starting around ten o'clock in the morning he begins to look forward to it. It's getting harder to imagine a day going by without it.

He's feeling a deepening sense of bitterness and frustration about his wife and family. He doesn't feel appreciated; if anything he feels that their insensitive demands only add to the burden. It angers him the way they seem to take the things his earnings purchase for granted. They've come to expect it as their due. It particularly enrages him when children put down his "materialistic middle-class trip." He'd like to tell them to get someone else to support them but he holds himself back. He tries to understand.

Coming home doesn't feel very comforting anymore, the way he thinks it should be. He doesn't sense any encouragement from the others and it bothers him that everyone just expects him to be strong all the time. He wonders what would happen if things fell apart and he couldn't play "strong man" anymore. It pains and irritates him just to think about it.

There's a growing gulf between him and his wife. She seems to have lost her vitality and tells him how tired and drained she feels. It's at the point where he resists sharing anything with her at all because he doesn't want to add to her burdens by laying his problems on her.

While in the first five or six years of marriage, she willingly played the role of comforter and "earth mother" to him, lately she seems to resent it whenever she feels that he relates to her like a "mother figure."

Maybe it's because that's the *only* way he seems to relate to her anymore. For example, their sex life is almost dead; it has become a chore to even get an erection. Most of the time he's just faking it in bed. He's had enough "failures" so that he begins to think that maybe he has one of those impotency problems. When he does succeed in the marriage bed it's often with a fantasy of another woman in his head.

Outwardly he's now the very model of a successful man—strong, self-contained, with a "normal," "happy" family. Inside however, he's struggling with powerful mood swings that he doesn't understand and can't control. When he feels high, he's really high, as if the sky were the limit. He feels powerful and he's in love with his life in those moments. Then he swings down and in these periods he feels depressed and paranoid about everything. Things seem futile, loveless, as if he were in a big cage with a bunch of trapped animals. The down moods come more often now and last longer.

The scariest part is watching what's happening to some of the guys he's known for the last ten years. Almost half are divorced and even though they talk about how happy they are to be free, they look lost. Besides, they gave up almost everything when they left their families and he feels scared and sorry for them.

Other guys who've stayed married are drinking heavily or look ten years older than they are. Everybody seems to have physical problems. If it's not an ulcer, it's a back problem. And all of them, including himself, are preoccupied with heart attacks. Besides cars and politics, a favorite topic of discussion at lunch seems to be diagnosing whether you're a Type A or Type B personality and how prone you are to a heart attack. Periodically he goes on an exercise kick but that never seems to last too long.

When he looks in the mirror he knows he's let himself go physically. But he rationalizes that anytime he wants to, he could get back into shape within a week or two. Every once in awhile, to prove that he hasn't lost much, he plays football or basketball with the kids, and he goes all out.

In between he gulps vitamin pills and takes other magic elixirs to slow down the aging process and to give him more time to get it together and enjoy the fruits of his success, which he still plans to do someday. But the signs he fears are staring him in the face every morning when he shaves. His face is fleshy, there's a puffiness under his eyes, and his hair is thinning and greying, almost by the day.

He's begun to have affairs. The first time he was really scared. He worried that someone would find out and the word would get out, of that he'd run into his wife as he was leaving the motel—even though it was miles from nowhere. She always seemed to have an uncanny sixth sense about where he was, even when he didn't tell her. He was afraid that she'd come driving by, see his car parked, and stand there waiting for him.

After a year of that he is more casual and careless about the whole thing. He even stops feeling guilty and tells himself he needs to do it in order to preserve his sanity. So that what began as an occasional, guilt-ridden experience is now a *raison d'etre*. He finds that it's the only thing he does during the week that he actually looks forward to and that makes him feel alive. He finds himself structuring his whole schedule around those few hours of sexual release and tenderness.

It's easier now than ever to hide his affairs from his wife because she thinks he's just about totally impotent and he's stopped trying to prove otherwise. So he doesn't even have to worry about whether he's got anything left over for her in the evening, after his afternoon flings.

In his isolation and alienation he becomes vulnerable to any woman who seems to reach out to him and show sensitivity to his feelings. Even a secretary who asks him how he wants his coffee and makes a remark about how tired he looks, turns him on and makes him feel recognized as a person with needs and feelings. With each new affair, though, he reassures himself that he's got everything under control. It's sex for sex sake and he'll never get emotionally involved, he tells himself.

That holds true for a couple of years and then he meets someone who seems different from the rest. She's in her twenties, and she seems vibrant, fresh, and unspoiled by life. Although she's young he sees her as someone who really "understands," someone who's mature, sensitive, and perceptive.

He opens up to her and tells her everything. She makes him feel free. The times that he's with her are rich and alive. Going to work every morning knowing she'll be there is like going to school used to be when he had a crush on a girl. He's careful about what he wears and how he smells.

Six weeks into the relationship and he barely thinks of anything or anybody else. When he's not with her, he's thinking about her. He never believed it would happen, but he's really struggling now with whether to walk away from everything and go off with her. Everything he's built up, his career, his family, his material possessions, all seem totally meaningless now, and he's willing to give them all up.

He's realizing in a powerul way that he wasn't getting any satisfaction from all of that anyway, so it's not *really* like he was giving up very much. He realizes now that they were all just props to protect him from his feelings and he feels sure that he could easily do without them.

Meanwhile, his girl friend tells him that she feels guilty and doesn't want to be a homebreaker and doesn't want him to leave his family for her. Yet when she tells him in the next breath she loves him, he's sure that she really secretly wants him to leave—even though she never comes right out and says so.

As the affair continues to become more intense, several things might happen. The first possibility is that his intensity, growing dependency, and almost frantic need for her might scare her and drive her away.

A second is that his wife might find out and after considerable hysteria and shouting at him to move out she tells him to give up his girl friend or she'll get a divorce. He has second thoughts and tries to break off the other relationship but he can't do without her for more than three days—he's hooked. He can't live without his girl friend. He moves out and divorce proceedings begin.

In all likelihood shortly after he moves out, he discovers

that his affair has already lost some of its excitement. He begins to wonder whether he used the affair just as a reason to escape. Maybe it was all a fantasy. He comes down from the energy high of his affair and he has a million doubts and second thoughts. He's given up everything he's worked for and he's beginning to wonder if he'd been going through some craziness when he left it all behind.

He tries for a reconciliation but it's very difficult. Whenever they get together she accuses him and he accuses her. All of a sudden his wife doesn't seem so fragile any more. She's hardened. She says she can't trust him and she tells him that he put her through too much torture and that she's tired of being a masochist. They go back and forth in dialogue for a while longer and then he realizes that indeed it is over. He salvages whatever he can. There's a good chance that he'll get deeply involved with the first woman who shows him compassion—not a twenty-year-old but someone closer to his age.

The third alternative is that he breaks off the affair in time, before his wife finds out. He's regained his "rationality." He tells himself that he was in a middle-age crisis, that he might be sorry for making radical changes.

So he goes back to his wife, but he begins to experience a deepening sense of depression, worse than he ever had before. He questions everything he put effort into all of these years, and it doesn't add up to much. He really works at slowing down. He tries to spend more time with his family. Sometimes everyone seems to be getting along and it makes him feel good.

Then it begins to grate on him. The kids have their own lives and don't seem interested in him anyway. His wife is complaining about physical symptoms a lot and when he takes her out somewhere, he can see that she's "trying" to have a good time and to stay interested but that she's really not. He himself knows that he's also trying too hard and is pretending to enjoy a lot that he doesn't really enjoy.

The extra time at home is making him restless. He realizes that leisure is not his thing. He can't see himself playing golf, reading, or watching television forever. He decides to get back into the old work routines. He never thought he'd feel this way but now he realizes that he'd almost rather be dead than face retirement.

The rhythm of life varies in smaller and smaller degrees. Sometimes it gets a little better, then a little worse. Maybe it stays the same for a while until there's another crises. All he wants is to keep his head above water. The success trip revealed itself for what it is.

9. The Lost Art
Of Buddyship

While preparing this chapter I kept thinking back to a recent ten-day seminar on aggression in which I participated. An actress conducted an evening program on the subject of aggression and the theatre.

She arrived early on the afternoon of the day of the program with a woman friend approximately her age who was helping her prepare for the evening presentation. Both are attractive, normal, equally successful heterosexual women and their friendship and interaction was very special to watch. Her friend hovered around her constantly, as involved and concerned that everything should be set up artistically and correctly as if the program was hers. She soothed and comforted the actress whenever she expressed any doubts or anxiety, constantly gave her encouragement, and communicated enthusiasm and excitement in anticipation of the evening. Then she helped her dress in an elaborate outfit, checking carefully to see that the make-up and the over-all look were just right. Forty-five minutes before the program was to begin she urged her to rest up and volunteered to get everyone seated and to inform them that there would be no smoking. Once it began she was there to participate and to help keep the program moving, and after it was all over she embraced her friend, helped her gather all the materials together and put them into the van. Along with a few others they went out to celebrate. Even though the woman friend was married and had children, she never expressed a feeling of being imposed upon nor rushed to get back home.

As I observed this interaction go on for seven or eight hours I was deeply moved, jealous, and saddened at the same time. The jealousy and sadness I felt was for myself and for many other men who I believe rarely, if ever, are capable of or experience such a caring, sharing, and loving relationship with another man—one in which great pleasure is taken in facilitating the accomplishment of the other, just as if it were happening to oneself. The existence of a "buddyship," in which they each facilitate and derive deep satisfaction from the success and achievement of the other, is uncommon.

I personally have to go back to my high school days to recall relationships of that nature—relationships where we honestly rejoiced in each other's triumphs. By the time I was in college it seemed that all of us men had already been thoroughly contaminated by the competitive posture that was subtly yet constantly undermining the possibility of genuine intimacy and caring. Instead, we were always checking each other out, looking over each other's women to see who had the prettiest, and never being sure if we could trust even our closest friends around an attractive girl friend.

It seemed like we all were hustling, and although we didn't want to see our friends fail, we also weren't very eager to see them do better than we did, to have them accomplish something of which we weren't capable. Then there was always the threat of being called a "fag" if one expressed affection openly to another male. When we saw such affection displayed we smiled at each other knowingly.

As adult males in our culture the phenomenon of being without even a single buddy or good friend is a common one—so widespread in fact, that it is not seen as unusual nor is it even spoken about. Rather, it is taken for granted. Many men I interviewed admitted to not having one intimate male friend whom they totally trusted and confided in. However, most of them seemed to accept this as being a normal and acceptable condition.

One weekend, while I was vacationing at a resort, I was discussing this book with the wife of a successful California real estate man. I mentioned that I was including a chapter on male friendships. She commented to me, "I wish I could find my husband a good friend. He's got loads of business acquaintances but not one real friend. And I know he's lonely. There's nobody he calls up for no reason except to say 'hello' and to chat. It's always a business or family thing."

At the time, this woman happened to be sitting with two women friends with whom she had come to the resort. Their husbands had stayed at home because of work commitments. Throughout the lunch they happily and comfortably chatted with each other, exchanging family anecdotes, discussing intimate matters relating to their husbands, mutual friends, the children, or themselves. They were clearly enjoying each other, listening and responding easily.

At a nearby table there were several men sitting together. In contrast to the women, they looked uncomfortable and strained. They seemed to have little to say to each other as they looked at their food or around the dining room for no one in particular. Occasionally, one would tell a joke or try to say something witty. The interaction was clearly tense until a woman came by who knew one of the men and joined the table. Suddenly the men became more animated and relaxed. Up until then there had been no dynamism in their interaction, no spontaneity and no relaxed sharing.

From both ends of the continuum, men seem to be blocked when they try to relate to each other. That is, they are not comfortable sharing their downsides—their failures, anxieties, and disappointments. Perhaps they fear being seen as weak, complaining losers or crybabies, a perception that threatens their masculine images. Neither do they seem to feel comfortable sharing their ecstasies or successes for fear of inciting competitive jealousies or appearing boastful. Consequently, verbal social interactions between men focus on neutral, largely impersonal subject matters such as automobiles, sports, and politics.

In the course of interviewing adult males I became particularly aware of the isolation of the married ones. While most denied being lonely, they almost all indicated that their wives were their only close friends, the only person they really trusted. They blamed the lack of male friends on the fact that they were too busy, but the real reasons were significantly more complex than that.

Until two years before I met him, Ralph, a thirty-three-year-old married glass salesman had one close male friend, an old, high school buddy. Then his friend began to make considerably more money than he did, remodeling his home and putting in a swimming pool and a billiard room. Shortly thereafter Ralph broke off the seventeen-year friendship explaining, "I didn't want him to think we were coming over just to use the swimming pool."

Where Ralph had been a vigorously independent and impulsive person before he married, he gradually became increasingly dependent on his wife, to the point that it scared and upset her. He told her that she was everything to him, and that he hoped he would die before her because he could never bear the loneliness of living without her.

Another example is Alan, aged fifty-four, the manager of a large travel agency. During our interview he expressed a sentiment that I had heard in various forms from many men. He said he didn't have any close male friends because the only guys he met were at work. "I avoid socializing with the guys who work for me. I think it's bad business. If you want to get the job done you've got to keep an impersonal kind of objectivity." He added that he really liked many of the men he worked with but he just couldn't take the risk of getting too friendly with them.

Alan could only think of one close male friend that he had had as an adult, and that person had died three years before. But as close as they were they only got together in the company of their wives. Whenever he called his friend on the telephone and spoke for more than five or ten minutes his wife would chide him for gossiping like a "washerwoman." This embarrassed him until the calls stopped altogether.

He finds it hard to make friends. Even though many of the men he meets are younger than himself he invariably relates to them in very competitive and defensive ways. He rationalized his lack of friends by the fact that his wife frequently complained of illness. "I'd feel lousy about myself if I went out and had a good time while she was sitting at home." Therefore, he spends his free time working on the cars, in the yard, or improving his home.

Gregory is a twenty-eight-year-old bicycle importer. According to his wife, Cindy, "Until Gregory got involved in group therapy, he didn't think another man would be interested in his feelings. He thought it was inappropriate to express feelings to another man." Before group therapy their friends were mostly Cindy's old girl friends from college and their husbands. The husbands never got together on their own, only as part of a couple.

Through group therapy Gregory has got closer to men but even so he tends to play the role of analyst to them and to listen rather than reveal himself. He noted that even in group therapy there was a lot of competition among the men, partic-

ularly about pinpointing feelings. "God help you if you aren't
in touch with your feelings first and best," he said.

Gregory still feels, however, that he doesn't have a "real
friend," someone he can confide in and completely trust. His
wife admitted that she puts a damper on some of his group
relationships because some of them have become too intense
and men would call Gregory for help during dinnertime or
very late at night. Gregory would always run out to meet
them if they wanted to talk and his wife began to resent this.

She also felt uncomfortable, however, about the fact that he
turned exclusively to her for comforting. "He'll tell me he feels
like a raw nerve and he wants me to comfort him, because
nobody else can. I rub his back and do my best to listen to
him. But he really gets furious when my mind wanders while
he's talking and I have to ask him to repeat his feelings."

Men who were interviewed rationalized their alienation
from other men in various ways. Other men were too "uptight," "fucked up," "defensive," "always competing," too
withdrawn," and "boring." As one said, "They're no fun to be
with. I'd rather be with a woman."

Married men often remarked that they didn't feel comfortable with divorced men because they claimed that it was too
depressing. They'd label the divorced man as immature. These
relationships, it often turned out, were also often discouraged
by the wife of the married man who was threatened by the
possibility that he would be influenced by his divorced friend.

Several divorced men commented that it wasn't until after
the marriage broke up that they realized that they had never
really enjoyed the company of many of the couples they socialized with during marriage. That is, many men who seemed
to enjoy each other's company when they got together as part
of a couple discovered that they had nothing in common when
they got together on their own without their wives.

Some men expressed the notion that if they burdened another man with their problems that this would obligate them
in the future. Friendships were seen, in a sense, as business
trade-offs. If you asked for help you would be expected to give
it at some future point.

In the area of friendship many men also related to their
wives as disapproving mother figures. They found it almost
impossible to indicate that they were going to spend an evening, day, or weekend with a male friend. Usually this was not

the case at the beginning of the marriage when the wives encouraged their husbands to have autonomous friendships. However, gradually this would change and in subtle ways the men began to feel that it wasn't worth the hassle of "asking permission" and of feeling guilty about leaving their wives at home alone with the children. They disliked having to explain what they did or said and who they had been with when they returned.

A friend told me of an instance in which he spontaneously invited another man to a poker game. The invited man became flustered and uncomfortable as he searched for an appropriate excuse that wouldn't make him look too henpecked. "I'll take a raincheck on that. I already told my wife I'd be home for dinner and she'd really be pissed off."

Because many married males work hard at maintaining the façade of a monogamous relationship, they are often fighting off the impulse to wander and to engage in casual sexual relationships. Because of these secret or repressed sexual desires they have chronically guilty consciences. Consequently, they expect that they won't be believed by their wives if they say they're going out with a male friend, particularly if they do so on a regular basis. They assume that they will be accused of having been with another woman or of having done something other than what they said they did.

Men married to women who play the traditional role of housewife and mother are particularly prone to feeling guilty if they enjoy themselves when their wives are at home. "It's not fair for me to be out having a good time, even if it's only with the boys, if she's at home with the kids." This same man might be very happy indeed if his wife went out alone with women friends. In a sense, by her doing so she could collect some trading stamps that would entitle him to a guilt-free time but alone at some later date.

Many men have come to view the need for a buddy as a remnant of inmaturity, or an adolescent need. However, their latent hunger for one is seen in their ecstatic response when they accidentally run into an old buddy. Often, it almost brings them to tears.

When two single men become friendly with one another their friendship frequently revolves around the joint pursuit of women. A friendship with no other reason than to enjoy each other's company tends to generate too much anxiety, particularly anxiety surrounding homosexual feelings and impulses.

The repression of closeness with one's own sex is not nearly as great in relationships between women and consequently they can comfortably be physical and playful with each other without anxiety.

In general, the extreme repression of male homosexual feelings in our culture and the intense anxiety about "being one" creates a major stumbling block in even normal male-male closeness. It results in the situation so commonly seen today where most adult men admit to being really comfortable only in close relationships with women. Getting close to another man, particularly if one does not have an equally close female in one's life, often mobilizes intense sexual anxieties, doubt, and suspiciousness. That horrible preoccupation of, "I wonder what he really wants from me" emerges as soon as an overture of warmth and friendliness is made by one man toward another.

A friend vividly recalled to me that in the middle of one of his European lecture tours his flight was delayed twelve hours due to engine problems. Each passenger was asked to share a room for the night with another passenger. My friend was booked into a room that had only one large bed. He remembered how careful he and his fellow male passenger were as they each slept on the very edges of their own side of the bed, in seeming terror of accidentally touching each other.

It is a tragic irony in our culture that men can only come comfortably close to each other when they are sharing a common target. As teenagers they come together in a gang or as members of a team out to "destroy" the other team. As adults, in wartime, they have a common enemy.

Many men recall their Army days as having been happy ones in the sense of their having felt real friendship or kinship with other men, an experience they have not had since. In the Army however, the common target was often the commanding officer, as well as the enemy. I am certain that POW's developed intense closeness as they joined together in the common pursuit of survival and hatred for their captors. The simple pleasure of being together with no other reason than to enjoy each other's company and support seems to be almost an unattainable experience for most men.

Because of the strong need to retain one's masculine image, men tend to be quite guarded around each other. Consequently, their talk rarely becomes personal. One man who was interviewed remarked at how amazed he had been when a male friend he thought he knew well separated from his wife. "I never even knew that they were having problems," he commented.

As an offshoot of women's consciousness-raising groups there have been efforts at creating male consciousness-raising groups. Reports describing the process of these groups suggest that there is a real struggle to keep them together. Group cohesion is tenuous and the interaction among the men tends to remain on an intellectualized, distant plane.

One man who had joined a male consciousness-raising group wrote about his experience. "In the world of men, I was alone, jealous, angry, untrusting, and uptight. Only with women could I let it hang out." While still part of his male consciousness-raising group, he contracted cancer. Before going in the hospital he received deep concern and warm support. Once in the hospital undergoing surgery however, there was not a word from any member of the group except one. "I knew the others all cared, but they didn't know how to handle it. This time I knew it was the group's problem, not mine. I was in bed but they were crippled. I felt disgust and sadness along with my anger."

I believe that these groups tend not to remain together for long periods of time because they lack a commonly shared target. In fact, attack or competition in these groups is tacitly and overtly considered taboo. Many men join them because they want to please their women or to learn how not to be male oppressors. Consequently there is a subtle group climate of self-hate and guilt induction. The target is oneself and each male is cautious about using words or relating in ways that are "typically male chauvinist." While there is mutual support to liberate oneself there is a dearth of joyful, playful, and unpremeditated ways of relating. Instead, a new subtle competition has arisen, competition to be the least competitive or chauvinistic.

The capacity for what I term "buddyship" is a genuine social skill, an area of competence that needs to be learned. I have chosen the word "buddyship" because of its connotations of youth and of spontaneity. This, combined with adult maturity contains the potential for the ultimate in masculine friendship. I have conceptualized four phases often present in the development of a buddyship. These four phases include the *manipulative* phase, the *companionship* phase, the *friendship* phase and finally, the *buddyship* phase.

The manipulative phase is where most relationships between men begin and remain. It is a phase of mutual using often to the benefit of both. It is also an interaction in which there is a mutually beneficial feed-off, such as occurs in the business world. The men come together because each has a skill, talent, or resource that the other can use. So long as the mutually shared goal exists and one man can help the other get ahead or expand his social or business territory, the relationship will remain viable. However, once there are no mutual benefits to pursue the relationship will tend to fade.

The manipulative phase may also assume other forms. A fairly common one is the relationship between the successful man and his "tag-along" or "kick me," the mentor and his student, the powerful man and his sycophant. The successful man is often a lonely, isolated person who can only relate comfortably with a person who respects, even adores him, and who is always available. The follower gets his payoff by basking in the aura of the other man, with the hopes that he will eventually make himself emotionally and actually indispensable (which often happens) and thereby reap some of the material and status rewards.

The manipulative phase can be destructive if one man is being used to his own detriment. In that case he is treated like an object and discarded when he no longer serves a purpose. The mutual caring disappears when the user has gotten what he wants and moves on to greener pastures.

The next step in the development of a relationship between men is the companionship phase. Companionship relationships are basically segmentalized ones which revolve around sharing a specific activity such as golfing, going to horse races, drinking together, pursuing women, playing cards, etc. If one of the men becomes ill, often he will not see his companion again until he has recuperated and is ready to play.

The mutually shared activity becomes the safe structure or excuse for getting together. It helps to define and limit the interaction in such a way as to make spontaneous intimacy unnecessary. Companionship is a form of mutual using but it is usually playful and benign. The relationship is limited again because there are no real roots of mutual caring. Consequently, when the commonly held interest no longer exists the relationship tends to wither and disappear.

Companionships, after a mutual testing period, may sometimes evolve into the friendship phase. One test of whether a companion can become a friend is the reaction to competition—winning and losing. If one man tends to incite the envy and jealousy of the other, then the friendship phase will not be reached. However, if the two men can find pleasure in teaching one another and in each other's individual success, a friendship can evolve.

In other words, a relationship can emerge from the companionship phase into the friendship phase, if each person feels included by the other, rather than extremely competitive. In this instance the alienating forms of competitiveness have been sublimated and the men do not feel beaten when they lose. The interaction does not generate a compulsive need to be better. There is pleasure in just being with the other and there is a capacity for a free flow of conversation, not necessarily confined to any one specific subject.

The friendship phase is one which involves mutual aid, compassion, and a willing readiness to be there in an emergency. A friend will lend money or other valued objects such as a car. He will inquire after his friend during illness and will provide a bed to sleep in when needed.

The friendship phase is relatively free of mutual manipulation, and more of the whole person is involved. It can, however, only become a buddyship once they have experienced a crisis that tests the friendship. If the crisis is transcended, vulnerabilities have been revealed and come to be respected, and deep trust has developed the buddyship phase can begin.

Buddyship is the deepest of male-male interactions. Buddyships, which already have endured crises, have rich dimensions that generally cannot exist even in the deepest male-female relationships. For example, it has facets of a good father-son and a loving brother-brother interaction. Each buddy, at alternate times, may assume the role of teacher or guide to the other and will revel in the other person's development and expanded skills. And there is also a sense of warmth and empathic understanding and comfort when one person is feeling weak, acting foolish, or being vulnerable. In these instances, one buddy gets stability and nourishment from the other. There is a happy, mutual sharing of resources, both material and emotional. The competitive element is inconsequential and a win for one becomes a win for both.

The brother-brother dimension of buddyship is one in which each looks out for the other, protecting him from exploitation. It is this phase of the male-male interaction that tends to be the most threatening to a wife or girl friend of one of the buddies. That is, a buddy will not hesitate to tell the other when he sees him allowing himself to be manipulated or self-destructively controlled by a woman.

Buddyship may also be threatening to an involved woman because many of its dimensions are not shared with her. Buddies will share deepest feelings about their relationships, personal fantasies, private or secret experiences. This may be very disturbing to an involved woman and her jealousy over the relationship may be deeper even than jealousy over a man's girl friend—partially because a relationship with another woman can be righteously attacked as being a betrayal of trust while a buddyship cannot.

Consequently, the woman may consciously or unconsciously attempt to undermine or destroy the buddyship. This may be attempted through derogatory comments, flattery, or suggestive innuendos. "What do you need him for? He's a big baby," "He just uses you," "You're like two overgrown adolescents," "He's not good enough for you," "He's jealous of you," "He's a loser," "You're always kissing his ass," "Why don't you go to bed with him? You spend more time with him than you do with me!" Suggestive remarks may be made implying latent homosexuality. Explosive arguments will occur particularly if a wife or girl friend sees "her man" do something for a buddy that he might not do for her or lend money or material possessions that she feels will cause her to be deprived in some way.

Female jealousy and resentment over a buddyship may also reflect her awareness that its roots may be deeper, because the relationship has more room for freedom, is less possessive, and does not have the components of jealousy and role rigidity that often exist in male-female relationships.

Buddyships are relatively role free. Each male feels safe enough to be open to act silly, stupid, and in spontaneous, child-like and affectionate ways which he may not feel safe enough to show anyone else.

The art of buddyship in our culture is undeveloped because

it requires time, a willingness to work through crises, to upset one's heterosexual partner, to endure hostile suggestions and innuendos about latent homosexuality, and a social maturity and competence that is not culturally recognized or rewarded the way that, for example, marriage is. If anything, a buddyship, if it is particularly intense, is embarrassing to others. Buddies are accused of delayed emotional development and of neglecting more important activities and relationships. Buddyships are often viewed as a threat to the "mature" husband-wife relationship because they require time, cultivation, commitment, mutual nourishment, and love. Their rewards, however, if achieved, are great because of their mutually supportive, nourishing, no-strings-attached aspects. They can endure stresses that few male-female relationships can because they do not have legal, contractual binds that force them to remain together.

The lack of such a relationship makes a man particularly vulnerable. It overintensifies his dependency on his woman, placing an emotional burden on her that can suffocate and destroy their relationship. Once a primary relationship with a woman breaks down the man has no one to turn to. In addition, once the male has totally and solely become reliant on a woman for the satisfaction of his emotional needs, he cannot afford to risk losing her. Consequently, he will be more prone to cling to an unhappy, unfulfilling relationship out of desperation and the frightening fear of being cut off from all emotional nourishment.

I believe that the lack of buddyship is also an important factor in the significantly higher male suicide rate and the significantly higher rate of death of divorced males as opposed to divorced females. Instead of reaching out for help, comfort, and nourishment from a buddy he hides behind a facade of strength and independence. Or he desperately reaches out for another woman, often throwing himself prematurely into another relationship. When no woman is available to him he may become engulfed in his isolation and alienation and become suicide prone.

It is my belief that the male needs to realize the importance of a buddyship relationship and learn to develop one. The path toward a buddyship relationship is a difficult and hazardous one that requires an awareness of the great need and survival value of such a relationship. It is much more difficult to

launch because while the male-female relationship tends to begin on the basis of a sexual attraction, the initial reaction between males tends to be one of cautiousness, anxiety about
openness and getting close, and some distrust. Therefore, while
a male-female relationship can arrive at a state of intimacy
fairly rapidly, the male-male relationship must endure various phases of development and be tested before the intimacy
of buddyship can be achieved.

The continuing impact of a buddyship is the development of
a deep mutual respect, trust, and pleasure in each other's company. Envy and competitiveness will increasingly recede into
the background while your buddy's growth and achievements
will begin to make you feel as good as if it were happening to
you. You will find growing interest in each other as total people and the specific things you do together will become significantly less important than the simple joy and comfort in being
with each other. A real buddyship will last a lifetime, remaining in the face of even massive personal changes in every
other aspect of life.

Guidelines Toward Achieving Buddyship

1. Begin by articulating those attributes which you respect in
   another man and those which you dislike.

   The positive attributes should include personality characteristics that generate joy, the freedom to be yourself, a
   willingness to open up and reveal yourself as a person, a
   sense of trust and safety, a desire to be talkative, humorous, and silly, an eagerness to explore, expand, and risk,
   and a receptiveness to learning new things when you are
   around that person.

   The negative attributes would include characteristics that
   tend to make you feel pessimistic, distrustful, guarded, inhibited, uncreative, bored, depressed, resentful, and scared
   about life when you are in that person's presence.
2. Draw a social nexus chart which pictures yourself in the
   center and the men that you consider potential buddies in
   circles around you. Place those you feel closest to nearest
   yourself and those you feel more distant from in circles
   which are progressively further away.

3. Now define in *specific* terms the characteristics you like and dislike about each. The following questions may be helpful to you in doing this:

   a) Is he guarded and secretive around me and do I feel guarded and secretive around him? In other words, do I feel like I'm prying whenever I ask him something personal? Do I feel anxious and regretful when I tell him something intimate about myself? Does he volunteer personal information about himself freely when he's around me and do I feel a strong desire to be open about myself when I'm around him?

   b) Do I feel comfortable calling him and would he call me up for no other reason than to say hello?

   c) Do I feel comfortable going over to see him on the spur of the moment, or do I feel I have to plan each meeting with him carefully and well in advance and only for a specific reason such as golfing?

   d) Do I feel respected and appreciated when I'm around him and do I respect and admire him?

   e) Do I have envious and competitive feelings toward him and do I sense that he has similar feelings toward me?

   f) Does he say and do things that embarrass me and do I seem to make him uncomfortable?

   g) Would I feel comfortable asking him to drive me to the airport, lend me his car, or give me a place to sleep when I needed that? Would I feel comfortable doing these things for him?

   h) Would I feel safe and confident if he were alone with my girl friend or wife and would I feel comfortable knowing that I could resist the temptation to seduce his girl friend or wife without his knowledge when he wasn't around?

   i) Do I feel I can grow, learn, and become more through a relationship with him and do I feel that I can provide the same kind of atmosphere and opportunity for him?

   j) Am I eager to know him as a total person or am I just interested in him to share a specific activity and would otherwise prefer not to get closer to him?

4. Once you have determined who is a potential buddy, recognize that two of the areas of greatest difficulty are those of trust and of dominance.

   To handle the area of trust ask your potential buddy to

define vulnerable areas with you; the kinds of behaviors that would destroy confidence and good feeling in both of you. Begin with the milder ones such as, for example, a show of indifference in him when you are discussing something of great importance to you. (One man mentioned to me his anger and diminished trust at a friend whose one ear was glued to the radio listening to a football wrap-up show while he was trying to discuss serious problems.) Then go progressively to the more sensitive areas such as making derogatory comments about you in front of close friends, not backing you up in an argument with others, revealing something personal to others which you had told him in confidence, or being seductive with a woman you care about.

To handle the issue of dominance, work toward equalizing power and decision-making so that neither of you winds up in the shadow of the other. Arrange tag-along meetings where one afternoon or evening you share in an experience of interest to him and then have him tag-along doing something which involves an area of your strength and interest.

5. Share your respective experiences of past disappointments and hurts in other friendships. Discuss incidents that have previously impaired or destroyed friendships for both of you as a way of learning about each other's areas of vulnerability and sensitivity.

6. Get together on a regular basis, perhaps once a month, a time specifically set aside to keep your relationship up to date and to avoid hidden injustice collecting. At this time discuss any incident or remarks that were made by either of you which caused disappointment or discomfort. In other words, be open with each other regarding areas of abrasion *before* they create great rifts.

10. Marriage:
Guilt By Association

A man's longing for a loving, intimate, exclusive relationship with a woman is powerful, contrary to the stereotype of him as strongly resistant to marriage and being "tied down." Men are marrying young—if not younger than ever before. Divorced men tend to remarry significantly sooner than divorced women. For the man in our culture, alienated from other men because of strong competitive conditioning and conditioned to relate to women manipulatively for sexual purposes, the craving for a special woman who is loving and understanding and who will recognize him as a person with needs is particularly urgent.

And yet something has been going wrong in marriage. The divorce statistics, which are staggering, are commonplace facts that almost everyone is familiar with. Those married couples who do manage to stay married for a lifetime may be confronted by their children telling them, "As partners in marriage and parenthood, your life is a lie. You betray yourselves, you betray us. Our family is turning into a tragic failure."[1]

According to one study of 601 couples who were asked the question, "Do you love your spouse?" only 11 per cent could answer unhesitatingly: "Yes."[2]

What are the roots of this dismal situation from the male standpoint?

In some cases the beginning of the end of the marriage, and of a young man's emotional integrity in that relationship, occurs on his wedding day when he experience butterflies in the stomach, a generally anxious and panicky feeling, and the impulse to flee. Since we live in a culture where men are taught to overcome reactions such as fear, the about-to-be-married male will be told that his frightened responses are normal and to be expected. Family and friends may give him subtly guilt-inducing interpretations of his inner experience, such as:

"You're afraid of closeness and commitment." "You're afraid to take responsibility." "You're afraid to give up your freedom." "You're reacting immaturely." Then he may be comforted with the reassurance that he will get over these fears and even will grow in the process.

Those guilt-inducing words "afraid of," which are often used to explain the male's resistant or negative reactions are a red flag, a battle cry which unfailingly strikes a responsive chord. They incite him to overcome, to prove himself, to accept the challenge, and to deny thereby the implicit demands of his feelings. From that moment on, as he strives to conquer and rise above his gut reactions of panic and resistance, instead of learning from the message it contains he is laying the foundation for the destruction of his marriage. These feelings of resistance that temporarily undergo repression may return in a flood sometime later when the marriage is on the verge of deteriorating or actually in the process of dissolution. Only then will he remember his early feelings and recognize the reasons for his original resistance. Until that time however, much of his energy will be spent in denying, overcoming, and rationalizing his feelings.

Just as he ignored his inner voice on his wedding day, he may continue to ignore it while he proceeds to try to make the marriage work. When he feels bored he will try to overcome it, or he will rationalize it away. When there is no sexual desire, he may become panic-stricken and begin to doubt his own sexual adequacy while he struggles to overcome his lack of sexual feelings. When he would rather not go home after work, he nevertheless dutifully goes, even though his resentment builds and he is withdrawn and uncommunicative when he arrives. During the day, he may telephone his wife from the office, because he thinks she wants him to, even though he may not want to. On weekends he will barbecue, run errands, do repairs, and sit passively in front of the television as he strives to fulfill the image of an involved husband and father. When he and his wife socialize with other couples, he will play the friendly host or charming guest, even when he is totally disinterested. So many of his responses will be motivated by his need to overcome, deny, and rationalize away his negative feelings that the marriage inevitably becomes so top-heavy with repressed emotion that it collapses. Only then does he allow his repressed resentment to come pouring forth. Until that time, however, he tends to engulf himself in self-hating accusations when he does not meet expectations and does not function or relate as he thinks he should. Self-insults such as, "You're a selfish bastard!" or "You're incapable of love," or variations on that theme become the nails which hold him in the marriage.

Rather than being a sign of immaturity or irresponsibility, the inner voice of resistance on his wedding day may have been a constructive inner prompting. This is particularly true for the young man. It is one of the male tragedies of our culture that marriage is condoned and sometimes even encouraged for a man in his early twenties—long before he has had time to develop and grow emotionally, to leave adolescence, to find himself vocationally and philosophically, and to achieve a fairly secure economic foothold. An early marriage may lay on him oppressive emotional and economic burdens that fixate him and trap him in a life-style devoted to the sheer necessity to survive, while aborting his personal and emotional growth.

From the standpoint of the male's early psychological conditioning, there seems to be too little foundation for achieving deep gratifications from marriage. In fact, a good case could be made that early male conditioning almost makes real satisfaction in marriage impossible. As a boy he is taught to achieve, to produce, to take on challenge, to conquer, and to explore. Unlike the little girl who may learn to find pleasure in playing house, being a mother to her dolls, and enjoying domestic games, rewards for such activities traditionally do not exist for the male. Whether these differences in early conditioning are good or bad, they nevertheless represent a psychological reality for the male in marriage.

Precisely because of these differences in gender conditioning, it is the man who so often finds himself falling short in his attempt to play the role of a mature marriage partner. He is often struggling to adapt to an environment and to live up to expectations not congruent with his early training or in keeping with his rhythm. He is pressing himself into a foreign mold. Consequently, he inevitably finds himself feeling like a spoiler and a depriver—the selfish one. In the eyes of others, he almost always emerges as the heavy. The often heard woman's complaint that it is she who is being exploited in the marriage is not wholly accurate. Undoubtedly, she has been limited by marriage, but it is the man's psyche that is particularly vulnerable. Because the male is not emotionally prepared for marriage, he is prone to deny and suppress his own identity and to fall into self-alienating patterns in his extreme effort to hold himself together in that relationship.

As an alternative to being booked on assault charges, Peter, age twenty-two, came for marriage counseling with his wife, Monica. Peter's vicious beating of his wife of one year had been interrupted by the police who were called in by frightened neighbors.

Peter was tall, muscular, and finely featured. His wife was a deeply tanned, classic beauty with long blonde hair and graceful, flowing movements.

Before they were married, Peter was sure he had found the ideal partner, a real man's woman. Monica shared his love for the outdoors. She enthusiastically joined him on dirt bike excursions to the desert. She happily clung to him on the backseat of his motorcycle as they raced down the freeways, and she took up surfing because she wanted to share Peter's love for the sport. Peter counted himself lucky to have found a woman who was the epitome of his image of femininity, but who was also comfortable and happy in his masculine world.

Shortly after their marriage Monica became pregnant and her attitudes started to change. Surfing, according to her, was adolescent, so Peter started going less often. Then she told him she was upset about his motorcycling. It was dangerous, and to prove it to him she would clip out newspaper accounts of motorcycle accidents and deaths and leave them on his pillow. Though Peter had never had an accident on a motorcycle he gave that activity up because he felt he owed it to Monica to stay healthy. Inwardly, however, he was becoming increasingly resentful and was beginning to feel betrayed by his wife's turnabout in attitude.

On a Monday morning Monica told him that she had plans to go out that evening with two of her former girl friends from high school. Peter, not expecting her to be home, without telling her went directly from his job to his friend's auto body repair shop where he planned to work on his automobile. He had the fender removed and was prepared to sand it down when he was called to the phone. His wife was angry. "Where are you? Where are you?" she screamed at him. In Peter's words, "I immediately felt guilty, even though I distinctly remembered her telling me that she was going out. I knew I had done nothing wrong. Still I was reacting like a bad boy. I kept asking myself if I had made a mistake and hadn't heard her correctly that morning.

"When I asked her what was wrong she said, 'Nothing's wrong except that I'm home and you're off playing with your car. Your car's apparently more important to you than I am.'" Peter tried explaining but Monica seemed too upset to listen. He told her he'd borrow his friend's car and be right home, to which she replied, "Don't bother," and hung up on him.

Peter was upset, complaining to himself, "That's not fair!" Nevertheless, he drove home anxiously. In the process of rushing, he was stopped for speeding and almost got into a fight with the policeman who seemed to Peter to be deliberately taking his time writing the ticket.

When Peter arrived home Monica was gone and he became frantic. He fantasized the worst, that she had run off and hurt herself. He felt overwhelmed with guilt, called her girl friends, and cruised the streets in his car trying to find her.

It wasn't until two-thirty in the morning, as he was on the verge of telephoning the police, that she came home. She had been with her girl friends at a nearby club and was a little drunk.

This time Peter became furious and began yelling, "Where've you been?" Monica's response was now mellow. She became loving and sexy when he saw how concerned he was over her. So she began to reach for him, saying, "I didn't think you'd be so upset. I told you I was going out with my girl friends."

She began to undress him and pull him into bed, but Peter was still so agitated and angry that while Monica was caressing and stimulating him, he pulled away from her. That triggered Monica. She lashed out, saying, "Why don't you go outside and make love to your car?" That ignited Peter; in retaliation he began hitting her until the noise and screaming got so loud that concerned neighbors called the police.

The interaction between Peter and Monica is a telescoped version of what so often happens to the once autonomous, "impulsive" male when he begins to adjust his rhythm to the needs of his wife. Gradually he gives up more and more things pleasurable and important to him. He reacts like a little boy when he thinks he's been caught doing something wrong. He turns his wife into a permission-giver and denies his own identity because he sees his patterns and interests as being unworthy or selfish.

While the build-up of underlying, hidden resentment and rage poured out suddenly and explosively in Peter's case, many other males simply express theirs unconsciously in the form of a passive and withdrawn retreat. In fact, this very pattern has become one of the most frequently heard complaints by psychotherapists from wives today. They say they feel starved out by the passivity and absence of communication from their husbands. This behavior on the part of the husbands is basically a safe, socially acceptable way of saying, "I don't want to be involved," without having to act upon this feeling overtly by leaving.

In Peter's case he had to reclaim his former interests and put himself first again before he could relate to Monica once more in a constructive, loving way. She began to see that she had been goading him on because, although she appreciated his devotion, she was unconsciously very threatened by the power she was developing over him in getting him to behave as she wanted. In a sense she was provoking him to test his limits and his ability to remain himself. She was quite relieved to see him take a stand even though it was a violent one.

Indeed, something awful happens to many men after they get married. As a sensitive and aware married woman I interviewed described the married men in her neighborhood: "They're all so passive. They have to hate their wives because those guys are hardly even people. A typical weekend day for them seems to mean trimming hedges, mowing the lawn, and puttering with their cars."

Furthermore, many married men seem to become progressively more childlike, dependent, and helpless in their interaction with their wives. Wives discussing their husbands with me in private often make comments such as, "He acts like a baby," "He's become so dependent on me it scares me. He won't do anything for himself," "He acts as if he's totally helpless," and "He's always hanging around the house and getting in the way. I wish he had some friends."

Many of these men ask their wives for permission whenever they want to do things on their own. When they describe the positive aspects of their marriage relationships it often sounds something like, "She lets me do things on my own and doesn't stay on my back, like a lot of other wives that I know." In essence, the wife has been given the role of permission-giver, or mother figure, by the male.

Progressively, the married man begins to distrust his own judgment and taste. He starts to believe that he is an unaesthetic clod who is only good in the business or working world and that his taste does not measure up to hers. Like mother, she knows best. As one real estate person expressed it to me, "I never sell to the husband. I always sell to the wife. If he likes the house it doesn't mean anything. But if she likes it, I've got a sale."

Because he is caught in a relationship that may not be intrinsically satisfying to him, although he is not always in conscious touch with his anger, resentment, and desire for autonomy, his negative feelings continually emerge indirectly in the form of passive-aggression. He is "in" the relationship but not "of" it. The passive expression of his frustration and discontent assumes many forms:

1) Extreme moodiness and occasional outbursts of rage that are precipitated by relatively minor things such as a misplaced sock, laundry done late, a button that hasn't been sewn on, a toy left on the floor, or a late meal.
2) Grabbing for the mail, a drink, and then hiding behind the newspaper or in front of a television set almost immediately after coming home from work.
3) Increasing expression of his wanting to be "left alone" when he's at home.
4) Increasing complaints of fatigue and physical ailments such as backaches, stomach aches, and headaches.
5) A drifting of attention when his wife is speaking to him causing him to ask her frequently to repeat herself, an indication that his mind is wandering and that he is not concentrating.
6) Having to be reminded constantly about the same things which he continually seems to forget, such as hanging up his clothes, taking out the garbage, etc.
7) A general resistance to talking about his day when he comes home in the evening.
8) Avoidance of sexual intimacy manifested indirectly by ei-

ther coming to bed after she's fallen asleep, or falling
asleep before she's come to bed. Other manifestations include bringing work home from the office and doing it
into the night, and staying up late to read or watch television.
9) An avoidance of eye contact with his wife.
10) An increasing tendency to confine his social life with his
wife to activities such as going out to eat or to a movie,
which do not require active interaction between them.
11) Generalized feelings of boredom. The boredom often disguises an impulse or desire to do things or be places other
than where he is. Since he is unable to own up to his real
needs he does nothing and sits home bored instead.

The passive-aggressive male is protesting in hidden, indirect
ways. Unable to assert himself openly or to own up to his
discomfort, his hidden resentment emerges in a myriad of underground ways. The message he is transmitting indirectly to
his wife is, "I'm afraid to do what I really want to do or to
express how I really feel, so I'll avoid feeling guilty by staying
at home. But you aren't going to get any satisfaction from my
presence either."

The actor-reactor syndrome is often a critical and destructive dynamic of male-female interaction in our culture, one
that is currently making it possible for the woman to label the
male "oppressor," "exploiter," and "chauvinist." As one
woman expressed it to her husband, "I was never allowed by
you to believe in myself as a first class, functioning person.
Men have an interest in preventing that."
Because he has traditionally assumed the active role, he also
automatically assumed the role of victimizer or "heavy." Because he fought the wars he was the destroyer while she was
the peaceful one. Because he assumed the primary burden of
economic survival, he also destroyed the ecology and was the
greedy, competitive one.
In the marital relationship, as in many other intimate male-
female relationships, the man almost invariably perceives himself as the "heavy," and can be perceived by the woman that
way also, for he has traditionally been the *actor*, while the
woman assumed the role of *reactor*. For example, he had traditionally been the primary provider. Consequently, if he

worked too hard or too long, she felt deprived and he felt guilty. If he was a poor provider, he felt inadequate while she could either assume a long-suffering role or berate him. If the children were having problems, she could blame it on his lack of active involvement and neglect. If the sexual relationship was poor, it was because he was too demanding, too quick, or too insensitive. Since he was traditionally the one who acknowledged and experienced his sexual desires more overtly, he was also more prone to "cheat." His wife, if she discovered him, could then react with outrage and hurt.

It is quite common, even in this day of more liberated sexuality for married men to express the feeling that, "If my wife ever found out that I was playing around on the side she'd leave me instantly." Nor is it uncommon for the wife who has never had an affair to react to her husband's "cheating" by leaving him and then sleeping with many different men in the first year, often in a spirit of justified retaliation.

Such was the case with Ron and Annie, who had been married for fourteen years and came for marriage counseling because they were on the verge of separation. According to Annie, the cutting blow that precipitated the marriage breakdown was that one year before she had discovered that Ron was having an affair with his secretary. She retaliated by having one of her own, now tearfully insisting that she didn't want to do it and didn't enjoy it (although the affair lasted two months) and entered into it only to punish Ron and to protect her own ego.

Ron was the "heavy." His affair had betrayed the trust in the relationship and was responsible for making her do something she said degraded her. It was, according to her, purely the self-protective response of a victim.

A recent research study on suicide is particularly instructive in defining the hidden lethality of this actor-reactor syndrome. The study pointed out that, in marriage, the suicidal spouse tends to see her or himself as self-effacing while the non-suicidal spouse sees her or himself as competitive and narcissistic. As the researchers pointed out, ". . . the tendencies of the non-suicidal spouse to seek only his own satisfaction are encouraged by the need of the suicidal person to have his desires ignored. In spite of the meshing needs that exist between the partners, the suicidal person often blames his suicidal behavior on his spouse's rejection of him."[3]

It is important to lay to rest this destructive actor-reactor, victim-victimizer syndrome and interaction, which results in the male carrying within himself a bottomless well of latent guilt which readily overflows. It is every male's responsibility to accept the total liberation of the female and to do everything he can to facilitate her emergence into an independent, openly assertive person in the male-female interaction. The traditional posture of the female in marriage as the exploited one is extremely hazardous to the emotional health and growth of the male, as well as the female. The model of a healthy male-female interaction in marriages of the future will be one in which each partner is directly assertive on their own behalf and assumes full personal responsibility for whatever happens to him. In other words, *he doesn't do it to her, but rather she allows it to be done to her because it somehow meshes with her needs,* and vice-versa. It is up to the female to recognize how her refusal to assert her needs directly and openly perpetuates the victim-victimizer syndrome.

There are many assertions about him that readily mobilize a man's self-doubts, self-hate, and guilt in marriage:

"You're afraid of intimacy and closeness."

"Why do you have to work so hard?"

"Can't you get more involved with the children?"

"Do you always have to stay glued to the TV watching sports?"

"Why don't you talk more? You never share anything, while I'm always telling you about myself."

"Why are you so cold and detached?"

"While you're running around enjoying yourself, I'm a slave to this house."

These accusations have a particularly harmful impact if the male believes that his response is his "problem." The male's behavior in these instances did not occur in a vacuum. Women have typically married men whom they could "look up to"—ambitious, self-contained, self-controlled, and success-oriented men. Soon after marriage however, they protest that these same men don't give enough of themselves emotionally. In effect, they are angered by the very characteristics for which they married them.

The following confrontation of a woman and her middle-aged physician-husband illustrates this phenomenon. She was largely attracted to him as a symbol of success and married him in part because he was a doctor. Approximately a year after marriage, however, she confronted him with the following: "You don't share of yourself, and I don't mean your damn money and position, your profession, the big-shot doctor. I'm sick of hearing about your goddamn office and about taxes and about problems with employees and patients and football games. You don't give of yourself to me, your *real self*."

Her physician-husband responded to this mainly with guilt. While he didn't understand what she meant by giving his "real self" because he thought that he had been doing that all along, he acknowledged that perhaps he didn't express his emotions enough.

Her protest, on the surface, had a reasonable ring to it. However, upon closer examination, it was as meaningless and destructive as if he had confronted her with: "Why don't you earn more money? You don't make any effort to gain position or power. All you've got is your goddamn feelings and I'm sick of hearing about your emotions. All you do is share of yourself. You never tell me about your achievements, drive, and success. I don't want to hear how you feel about this or that. Make something of yourself in the outside world."

Society has placed confusing expectations on the married male, demanding that he be all things to all people: the capable provider, the aggressive competitor, the wise father, the sensitive and gentle lover, the fearless protector, the cool, controlled one under pressure, and the emotionally expressive person at home. Because he is unaware of the inherent contradictions in these expectations and is out of touch with his true capacities and needs, he has accepted the idealized image expected of him and is destroyed in the process of trying to live up to the impossible. He will need to approach marriage with more objectivity, making certain that he will be getting as much out of it as he is giving up for it. While the woman is beginning to throw off her traditional modes of responding and performing it is the male's responsibility to establish new modes for himself, modes that will provide for his growth, comfort, satisfaction, and an opportunity to live in flow with his own rhythm.

More than anything else, he must see beyond the accusation of "male chauvinist," which only serves to mobilize his guilt and paralyze him, and instead he must create a marriage style that is truly compatible with his individual being.

The new definition of marriage for the male will only emerge once he has recognized and translated his often passive-aggressive marriage style into direct, open feelings of self-assertion. Only then can he develop a new, self-enhancing, direct, and honest way of relating.

Fathering

"Mommy, if the doctor brings the baby in his bag, and if Santa Claus brings us toys; if God will punish me when I am bad, and if money grows on trees, why do we need daddy?"[4]

Psychological and medical studies have indicated that young men often report headaches, nausea, indigestion, backaches, and the beginning of ulcers during their wives' first pregnancies. In addition, the arrest rate for sex offenses such as child molesting, masturbation in public, attempted rape, and the making of obscene phone calls is apparently significantly higher for expectant fathers.[5]

The traditional explanation for this phenomenon is that the expectant father is behaving regressively under stress. It is my belief, however, that these symptoms may also represent an unconscious protest, a desire to flee from the responsibilities of fatherhood—feelings that the male did not allow himself to experience consciously and take responsibility for before his wife's pregnancy.

Just as about-to-be-married men strive to overcome their resistance to marriage, many young men are also unable to consciously own up to their resistance to fatherhood. They impregnate their wives and later develop disturbing psychological or psychosomatic symptoms.

Men who are emotionally upset during their wives' pregnancies may be told by professionals that they have an underlying fear of being replaced by the child as their wife's favorite love object. The wife is given well-intentioned advice, such as: "By indicating her belief in her husband as a man, as a human being, as well as a prospective father, the pregnant wife may be able to allay any fears he may have that he will be replaced in her love by the unborn child."[9]

In effect, the prospective father is being portrayed as a child himself, competing with his own child for "mommy's" love. If this conjecture is indeed true, it only further suggests the immaturity of too many men who become fathers.

There is a widespread cultural notion that it is better for a man to have children when he is still young, energetic, and not set in his ways. In fact, many young couples see parenthood as a form of paying their dues or getting a responsibility out of the way. The rationalization is, "If we have them now, then when we're in our forties they'll be all grown up and we'll still be young enough to enjoy ourselves and do the things that we *really* want to do." Clearly, the process of raising children is seen as an obligation—like military duty or paying taxes—to be gotten out of the way so there'll be time and money left for the more pleasurable things.

Fathering before he is ready is one of the more self-destructive ways the average man aborts his own growth and development. In a moment of sentimentality over the idea of becoming a father, some young men lock themselves into financial binds and emotional demands that drain their energies and resources psychologically and materially. Unconsciously, they may be fathering out of one or more of the following reasons:

A public affirmation of his potency and his manhood: Fathering a child is a way of offering concrete proof to the world that he is able to have an erection and to impregnate a woman.

A "Please Mommy" trip: For the mother-bound male, fathering a child may be a way of pleasing his own mother. It is proof that he is mature, willing to take on responsibility, and he fantasizes that it will make his mother happy to be a grandmother.

Career and image reasons: To the career-oriented, upwardly mobile male, having a baby will lend to his image of "maturity," "responsibility," and "stability." He believes that he will be looked on more favorably by his employer and may be more likely to be promoted now that he has offered visible proof that he is a settled married man and not a playboy.

To prove to his wife that he loves her and is committed to the relationship: This is perhaps the most common motivation of all. He has a child because he wants to make his wife happy and to help her fulfill herself as a woman, or so he believes. In many such instances, the male discovers only too late, usually as the marriage is breaking up, that his wife resents the responsibilities of being a mother and sees her children as a burden, rather than as a pleasure. With increasing frequency, the contemporary woman is even becoming agreeable to giving up her children after divorce.

Security: He feels that having a child will cement the relationship. Particularly if he is insecure in the marriage he may father a child because he believes that his wife will then be less likely to leave him.

The fantasy of immortality: The desire to have a son is often tied in with the desire to have someone who will carry on the family name. In addition, it is a way of leaving behind concrete proof that he was alive. Having a child is unconsciously the best way of insuring his immortality.

Something for my old age: This motivation involves the belief that having a child will prevent loneliness in his old age. Perhaps there is even the fantasy that his children may someday take care of him when he is unable to do so himself.

Children as indirect aggression targets: He may unconsciously have children to serve as indirect aggression targets, taking the heat off the relationship. In these instances, children become outlets for the anger and frustration that exists between husband and wife. Children also may be used as blame targets for the unhappiness within the relationship and may serve as distractors from the boredom of deadness in the marital interaction.

Relieving self-hate: The man who has a tendency to label himself as selfish, immature, and narcissistic if he indulges his own pleasure and freedom impulses, is reassured by becoming a father that he is not these things and that he is capable of being concerned for someone other than himself.

The above reasons are not to imply that fathering is always based on fantasy-oriented, self-destructive motivations. However, many men who father, whether young or old do so for the wrong reasons. There is, I believe, in this day and age where children do not necessarily enhance the survival potential of the family, only one "right" reason for a man to father children, and that is that the *process* of being a father excites him and is seen as enriching, fulfilling and joyful, and the realities of his life allow him to participate fully. However, few men have reached that level of maturity before they have undertaken this critical and difficult responsibility. Having children should be saved for last, for the time when the man has played out his fantasies, has had relationships with many women, explored and given himself the gift of finding out who he is. The time that he can anticipate having children with the same enthusiasm as he might, for example, anticipate going to bed with an appealing woman, is the time to become a father. *Only such a driving motivation, I feel, justifies undertaking the heavy responsibility of fathering and will result in a genuinely positive orientation.*

A recent study by a University of California sociologist who compared men who fathered early to those who first became fathers at an older age, disclosed that it was the young fathers who experienced "role strain and discomfort" about parenthood. The older fathers were "significantly more self-possessed and comfortable. . . . Parenthood to these men was something like a benevolent trusteeship, their function being one of promoting the autonomous development of their children, rather than shaping them." Young fathers were seen as more concerned with "competing family-and-career stage demands, economic pressures and so on. . . ."

Successful fathering is not a matter of education or the learning of techniques. Rather, it is a matter of being fully conscious of and fluid with one's inner emotional responses and secure in one's own judgment. There is no impulse to take a backseat role and defer to the greater wisdom of the "maternal instinct." This kind of male will have already learned how to trust and respect himself and will have overcome the cultural stereotype of the young father as a bumbling clod who does his job best by staying out of the way.

In general, it is time for the male to totally reevaluate his orientation to marriage and fatherhood. The female has set the stage and facilitated the process by allowing herself to emerge honestly as a person—refusing any longer to confine her role simply to that of devoted wife and mother. She even has had the courage to disavow the hallowed notion of the "maternal instinct." It is time for the male to own up likewise.

On The Right Of The Male To Determine His Future As A Parent

Now that women are no longer victims of oppressive laws that denied abortions to them, paternal responsibility without the consent of the father is a sexist relic.

Now, the woman retains the ultimate legal right to decide on all matters of childbirth. If she becomes accidentally or unexpectedly pregnant and wants to have the baby he cannot say "no," and demand an abortion. In spite of this lack of decision power, he still retains paternal responsibility financially and legally.

On the other hand, if the father wants the baby and the woman wants to have an abortion he again cannot impose his will, even if he agrees to assume full responsibility for the child.

I propose that any couple intending to have a child sign a contract formalizing this mutual desire. In the absence of such a contract the male must be given the prerogative of demanding an abortion unless he is released from any financial or legal responsibility if the woman insists she wants the child despite his request to terminate the pregnancy. Otherwise whenever birth control measures fail the male becomes a potential victim because he is legally responsible without having made the decision to have a child.

It is, I believe, a form of discrimination for the male to be held responsible for an unplanned child while the woman is permitted to decide whether or not she wishes to have the baby.

Guidelines For Marriage And Fatherhood

1. Before marrying probe your inner experience and openly acknowledge and explore any inner resistance, commonly known as prewedding day panic. Do not simply strive to overcome these hesitations, but rather try to learn from them. They preserve growth and may help you avoid making a complicated and self-destructive mistake.
2. Once married, trust and be open to your inner responses to your life situation. Do not reject, hide, or try to overcome feelings of boredom, the desire for greater autonomy, or sexual resistance to your mate. They are your truthtellers and the suppression of them will thoroughly contaminate the relationship with hidden aggression and lay the groundwork for total marital alienation.
3. Refuse to accept labels such as "selfish," "inadequate," or "immature." They are only guilt-makers that will distract you from discovering what you really feel. At the same time, do not assume roles and postures that are onerous to you in order to prove that you are not any of these things.
4. Avoid placing your wife in the role of permission-giver. She is not your mother and you are not her little boy. You are free to do what is important for you to do in order to fulfill yourself as a person.
5. Learn to recognize, respect, and hold on to your own taste and sensitivities in clothing, furniture, housing, and friends, etc. They need to be preserved in order for you to maintain your own identity.
6. Have children for the expectation and anticipation of the joys of the *process* of being a father. Do not have them if you are too busy to participate in their rearing or expect to take a backseat to the wisdom of the "maternal instinct."
7. As a general rule, put yourself first, except for those occasions when you genuinely want to make your wife's needs

primary. Assume the risks of owning up to who you really are, completely and joyfully. Remember that you are not the "heavy" whenever you cannot comfortably wear the traditional mantle of the married male.

11. Divorce:
The Penalties For Leaving

Perhaps the best thing about a divorce is that for the first time the man is forced to look at his wife more as a total person rather than as a projection of his fantasies. The awakening is rudest for the more rigid, role-oriented man who has imagined himself as a super-protector and provider and his wife as a selfless, helpless, and unworldly being.

During a divorce, it is not uncommon to see even the seemingly most docile of women become canny, aggressive opponents. She may behave that way directly on her own behalf or she achieves the same result by hiring a hard-nosed attorney to do battle for her. In the latter instance she can disclaim personal responsibility for any of the lawyer's demands.

Typically, during divorce there is an outpouring of long-suppressed rage on both sides. The difficult lesson to be learned is that the seeming transformation of feelings from love to hate or attraction to revulsion that occur during this period is not merely a product of divorce acrimony, nor indicative of sudden change. Rather, the divorce process itself simply triggers the surfacing of dormant, underlying feelings that have been kept repressed as the inevitable result of the romantic, illusion-filled approach to courtship and marriage in our culture. This orientation is one in which husband and wife need to see each other in mainly positive ways while avoiding confrontation over negative feelings, conflicts, and threatening concerns. Consequently, when they are finally expressed they emerge in a torrent of uncontrollable, severely alienating hostility.

Dr. George R. Bach, with whom I often conduct Pairing seminars designed to facilitate more authentic communication for single people, once commented in a humorous vein during a lecture that the quietest place in America is the dining room of the Niagara Falls honeymoon lodge. The newlyweds gingerly tiptoe around each other, determined to avoid any conflict or negative exchanges.

This distorted cultural orientation to aggression is discussed in the book I wrote with Dr. Bach entitled, *Creative Aggression*. It describes the processes and forms of blocking out the recognition and expression of negative feelings among intimates and the destructive, inevitable consequences that result.[1] The male in love, for example, is bent on perceiving his woman as being totally different from all other women. He tends to see her as devoid of aggression, particularly toward him. It is not uncommon for brothers, sisters, parents, and friends to see the negative side of a woman that her lover or husband-to-be seems totally oblivious of and even tends to deny ("They don't understand her," "They don't know her like I do.") until the marriage is in the process of breaking up.

Usually only during a divorce can husband and/or wife acknowledge that "I have nothing to say to him (her) at all. We get together and we just kind of stare at each other. Or we wind up accusing each other and dragging skeletons out of the closet." One woman, in describing the experience of being touched by her ex-husband, commented that she felt like she was being rubbed by sandpaper. A recently divorced man remarked that he literally became nauseous at the thought of making love to his ex-wife. These were, in part, long-suppressed feelings emerging full blown now that it was permissible to feel them. (Imagine a husband or wife expressing these feelings to each other while they *still* were married.) Only during divorce do the individual partners allow themselves to become aware of all the ways in which they had shut out the frustration, boredom, and resentment.

Even feelings of total estrangement, as if one's spouse had never even existed are not uncommon. These reactions only point up the extreme repression of feelings and the gross denial and numbing of emotions that cause relationships to become so top-heavy with unreality that they inevitably collapse. The same things that were formerly experienced as "good" and "beautiful" *during* the marriage are now seen as "bad" and "ugly" once it has ended. The physical attraction that was there becomes a feeling of not even wanting to be touched at all. The deepest understanding becomes a total lack of communication and the greatest love and devotion is transformed into intense antipathy.

The formerly "nicest" couples often have the most vicious of divorce experiences. The woman who viewed her husband as a complete "nice guy" is just as vulnerable to shock as the man who perceived his wife as an all-loving, devoted "earth mother." The "nice guy" is suddenly cold and uncaring and "earth mother" is suddenly heard wishing her ex-husband dead.

Male Self-Destructiveness In Divorce

Whether the man initiates the divorce or is the one who is left, male self-destructiveness is often affecting his behavior during a divorce.

When the male initiates the breakup, he tends to engage in self-punishing behavior as acts of retribution and to assuage his guilt for having been the "villain." He is prone to paying his dues by making grand, impulsively generous gestures. This is frequently the case when there is another woman involved and he has initiated the separation. He will, in a moment of romantic omnipotence and guilt inform his wife that, "You can have anything you want." Feeling temporarily liberated and powerful he rationalizes: "I can start all over again. Besides, I'm through with the middle-class materialistic trip. I'm finding out that those things really don't matter and I'll never do that again anyway."

In this way he also reassures himself of his fairness. His grand gestures allow him to feel he is still the good chum, the responsible and the concerned protector of his family. Since they can't have him anymore, they can have almost everything else. He can walk away from his empire because he has found himself and therefore nothing else really matters.

The affair that liberates him from the marriage may prove to be short-lived. Reality pounds these romantic illusions more harshly and quickly than it did in his marriage. Ultimately, he may discover as many do that the affair was simply an excuse, a lever with which to extricate himself.

When his affair is in jeopardy he may experience regret and doubt and begin to make overtures to his wife for a reconciliation. He may be stunned to discover how quickly the wife he thought he had destroyed has found her strength. After her initial reactions of shock and hurt she often experiences her own deep sense of relief and freedom. She surprises herself discovering how much she enjoys her time alone and the new social life she has begun and she may be totally disinterested in the idea of a reconciliation.

In effect, what is happening is that, by leaving, the husband has done the dirty work for both himself and his wife. While he has assumed the role of rejector and marriage destroyer, he has actually released himself and his wife from a marriage that on some level was equally uncomfortable for both of them.

As the *actor*, the man made the first move and therefore assumes the blame. In addition to paying legally in many states for being at "fault," he also pays with guilt. His wife, on the other hand, by being the one who has been left, can guiltlessly and righteously walk away with the reassuring satisfaction that she was not responsible. Furthermore, she can comfortably feel, if she wishes, that she owes him no kindness because he betrayed her.

The feeling of guilt for leaving is one trap from which the liberated male *must* free himself. In every marital relationship the behavior of one person is in large part a result of the marital interaction. No behavior emerges strictly out of context of this interpersonal relationship. This is a lesson which the male must learn. Once he has assimilated that awareness, he will be less prone to engage in self-destructive, undoing behavior in order to release himself from guilt.

The man who leaves is more likely to have a woman waiting in the wings for him than vice-versa. In part, this again reflects what I believe to be his deeper dependency needs and his fear of being alone. This notion seems to find some corroboration in the statistic that shows that the divorced male remarries sooner than the divorced female.[*]

There are other factors that might explain this phenomenon. The male who leaves is also often devoid of any other supports and is therefore more urgently in need of nurturance. Typically, when he leaves he loses his home, his children, and many of the friends they shared as a married couple. Typically, the divorcing male has no close male friends to turn to either.

The nature of his relationship with his parents and siblings makes it difficult and embarrassing to ask for help. His image as a man would be threatened and he needs to project himself to his family as strong and independent. The masculine posture that prevents him from seeking help, expressing weakness, or vulnerability, and leaning on someone else intensifies his isolation and the need for another woman to replace his wife, even before he has made the break with her.

Women seem able to initiate the breakup of a marriage more easily—whether or not there is another man involved. They can end the relationship simply because they feel unfulfilled, stagnant, or degraded by their role. The trauma of leaving is softened because they tend to have more capacity to accept emotional support and nourishment from friends and family during this time of crisis.

During the last decade, the initiation of a separation or divorce by the woman has, in fact, become an increasingly common phenomenon. This is one of the most dramatic reversals in the male-female relationship in our culture. The male, in these instances, is often totally disbelieving and unprepared. Being abandoned by his wife never even seemed to him to be a remote possibility.

The impact is therefore particularly devastating. He often engages in excruciatingly humiliating manipulations to try to win her back. In the process, terror, panic, and depression may put him on the brink of suicide. Severe mood swings may continue for many months and will be interspersed with fantasies of violence toward his rejecting wife and her lover, if one exists.

Particularly vulnerable to emotional devastation is the man who was unable to perceive his wife as a person with needs and feelings beyond the superficial trappings of her role as wife and mother. Donald M., an engineer in his thirties, was a classic example of this as he passed through distinct phases during the divorce process.

Donald was ambitious and business-oriented. Along with two partners he purchased a factory approximately three hundreds miles from his home and went into computer parts manufacturing shortly after his marriage to his wife, Kathy. This meant being away on business at least twice a month.

His wife had been raised in a strict, moralistic family. Donald married her when she was twenty-two-years-old and he was the first man to sleep with her.

Kathy fulfilled Donald's fantasy of a good wife and mother.

Therefore, it hardly bothered him that she was almost totally unresponsive sexually. She complained that having sex was physically painful. She visited a gynecologist to determine if there were physical causes for her pain. The doctor informed her that the problem was not physical and that as soon as she learned to relax the pains would go away and she would begin to enjoy sex.

In some ways Kathy's discomfort with sex was even reassuring to Donald. To him it meant that she was a traditional old-fashioned woman. Indeed, he might have been more concerned had she been overly responsive sexually. This way he could comfortably rationalize going away on his business trips without feeling that he was depriving her, and he didn't have to worry that she might be unfaithful to him.

While Kathy secretly felt frustrated sexually she avoided discussing this openly with Donald for fear of threatening his male ego. Rather, she preferred to go along with his fantasy by pretending that sex was unimportant to her. Unconsciously it also gave her some control over him. Because of her pain during intercourse she could make him feel that each such encounter was a sacrifice and a love token which she granted him and for which he should be grateful.

They had two children in the first three years of marriage. As the business grew, Donald would be away from home for progressively longer periods of time. Though Donald often felt frustrated sexually, going to bed with other women was unthinkable. He couldn't do that while she was sitting at home taking care of their children and being deprived of his presence.

Kathy meanwhile became increasingly resentful over being left at home alone. She hesitated sharing these feelings with Donald because she couldn't see a solution. The family needed the money. Instead, after eight years of marriage she began to feel she was entitled to have an affair.

Her first affair lasted only three weeks. But in it she discovered that she was very sexual indeed. There was no pain. Her married lover was erotically aggressive and Kathy found herself doing and enjoying things she never imagined she could. She discovered that she was even turned on by oral sex, something she always had reacted to with disgust when Donald suggested it.

Shortly after the affair ended, she began another one. Donald did not know what was going on. He was busy with his own work and oblivious to Kathy's preoccupation and emotional distance when he was home.

At the time when Donald's business was at a peak and when everything seemed to him to be going beautifully, Kathy announced that she felt troubled and unhappy with their marriage and needed time to be alone to think things over. She asked Donald to move out. When Donald protested, she blamed him for devoting more time to his work than to her, for ignoring her, and for being cold and selfish.

It hit him very hard. He had not seen any warning signs. He reacted disbelievingly and urged her to get psychiatric help. He blamed it all on her emotional problems. Kathy promised to go for help but only after Donald moved out. When he resisted, she threatened divorce. In his desperation to keep her he agreed to leave.

Donald had begun the phases common to many men whose wives unexpectedly announce their decision to leave. The first phase was a reaction of total disbelief and protest.

In the second phase, Donald assumed a beaten dog look and a disconsolate willingness to accommodate by being a "nice guy." He felt sure, knowing Kathy as well as he thought he did, that she would recognize his suffering, feel sorry for him, and ask him to return. He accepted in total faith her assertion that she needed only a little time to think things over. So he rented a small apartment.

Three months passed and there was still no way he could pressure Kathy to take him back. Whenever he tried to she would counter that she still wasn't ready and that if he couldn't understand it might be better to divorce.

Another two months passed and Kathy was still no closer to being "ready." At this point Donald entered the third phase. He began to take all the blame for the breakup and promised to go into therapy himself to change and become a better, more involved husband. Session after session Donald accused himself to the therapist, often echoing Kathy's contentions. He had been selfish, cold, a disinterested father, and had also treated her chauvinistically.

He would repeatedly beg the therapist to tell him how to get Kathy back. He would plot strategies and search for the magic words that would convince her to return. All along he insisted to his therapist that he was certain there were no other men involved in Kathy's life.

Several months went by and Kathy decided it was time for a divorce. However, she was reluctant to confront him directly. She felt protective of him and didn't want to see him hurt. So she told him she thought they ought to see his therapist together. Donald was elated, certain that this meant she wanted to work things out.

During the session the therapist commented that Kathy seemed very remote while Donald was going through emotional hell. At that point she acknowledged that she had no energy left for the relationship and wanted out.

Donald entered the fourth phase. The phases of denial and hope were over. His worst nightmare had become a reality and he showed early signs of a breakdown. He cried, trembled, and for several weeks was nearly immobilized. He would call Kathy four or five times a day under any pretext, then plead with her to reconsider. He would cruise around the city in his car for hours and invariably wind up circling their house.

He couldn't concentrate and he couldn't work. In fact, he felt revolted by his business, blaming it for destroying the only thing in his life that had given him meaning. He continually replayed old family scenes, trying to understand how it had all fallen apart.

After two months of this hell he began to pull himself out and entered the fifth phase—social and emotional reemergence. This phase is different for different men. In Donald's case he started dating and soon met a divorced woman two years younger than himself. She gave him comfort and understanding and in a short time they were living together.

In some other instances, as the rejected husband begins to regain strength and frees himself from his emotional investment in his ex-wife, she may regain interest and make reconciliation overtures. By now she may have acted out her own fantasies and may have found them wanting. Her husband, who no longer is groveling is now also more attractive to her. The husband, though insisting he's through, may begin to waver. He feels torn again and may even feel guilty for not responding in the loving way his wife seems to want him to.

The experience of most men in the divorce process puts the lie to the myth of male autonomy, independence, and strength.

Whether he leaves or is left, the divorce is shattering and guilt-inducing. When he is the rejected one he is often left dazed, disbelieving, and desperate. He may rage like a baby from whose mouth the breast has been prematurely removed. Eventually, like a severely rejected infant, he may even withdraw into an apathetic, detached, and low energy stupor.

One recently returned POW from the war in Vietnam, whose wife divorced him after he returned from years in a prison camp, indicated that he found that being in prison all those years was far less painful than going through the divorce when he got home. "In prison I could take the physical pain. I lived eight years on crutches because I broke my right lower leg in two places when I bailed out. I was tortured like the other POWs and I found I could stand that. But the emotional test of the past few weeks has been hard to pass," he said.[3]

The man who initiates the divorce is equally as conflicted; he is submerged in guilt for having been the aggressor, the spoiler, the selfish one. Typically, the man feels responsible, whether he leaves first or not. When she leaves him he blames it on his lack of sensitivity to his wife's needs or his preoccupation with work, etc. When he leaves he feels guilty over being the villain.

Historically, the legal system has taken a similar view. Divorce proceedings were generally designed to punish the male who in most cases was seen as responsible for the marriage breakdown. Whether because of circumstances or as a courtesy, the bulk of divorces were filed by women. The reason the male was typically the one served with the papers was that the "accused," the one "at fault," stood to be punished by the court. Prior to "no fault" divorce laws which have been enacted recently in some states, only the party against whom the divorce was granted could be compelled to support the other.[4] Before these new laws, if the man, for example, was found guilty of committing adultery, he was automatically punished by having to give up more than half of their community property to his wife. Sometimes this amounted to as much as 75 per cent of the property or more.[5]

The greatest tragedy for the man in a divorce is that he is often brought full circle back to where he started or worse. He may be forced to give up almost all of what he spent years building up. As one divorced man described it: "I'm stripped.

Everything I put together for fifteen years is gone."⁹ A blue collar worker mentioned that after twenty years of marriage, all he had left was his car and his clothes when he divorced. He rationalized, "Even though I lost everything I worked for in twenty years at least I'm not a slave anymore."

The divorcing man with children stands to lose his home, many of the things in it that he loved, much of his property, a significant portion of his income, and he may find himself progressively alienated from many of the friends he socialized with as part of a married couple. And he may virtually lose his children, if not in immediate fact, then as the inevitable long-range result of being an absent father.

A divorced woman who had remarried two years after her first son had been born, remarked of the ex-husband with whom she had the son, "He makes my life miserable because he won't let go of our son. He still insists on seeing him every weekend."

Her remark represents in the extreme a very common attitude. Once divorced, if the wife has custody as has traditionally been the case, the children increasingly become her property. The woman who remarked about her husband's not letting go had two more children by her second husband. Her ex-husband was now a distant, annoying relic of what she viewed as being an unhappy past. She considered her present husband the father of all of her children.

Still another divorced woman, angry because her ex-husband had made some bad business deals that caused him to be two and a half months behind on his alimony payments, remarked that she would simply forbid him to see the children until he had made the payments. The unspoken implication is that the children belong to her and her ex-husband has to pay for the privilege of his visits.

Research has indicated that a woman who remarries tends to experience growing negative feelings toward her former husband as she unfavorably compares her previous marriage to her present happier one.⁷ Inevitably therefore, she will encourage the children to attach themselves to their new father.

The reality is that a divorced father who does not have custody becomes increasingly more estranged from his children. If his ex-wife remarries, his role may be taken over by his ex-wife's new husband.

It does not require great sensitivity to understand the agony of a divorced father whose children are now calling their mother's new husband or boyfriend "Daddy!" If mother moves out of the area or state, or if out of economic necessity father is forced to relocate, that may virtually spell the end to the relationship with the children. In the course of such long absences, the children out of emotional self-defense may begin to repress his memory or even come to dislike him in order to feel more comfortable about his absence.

Consider the anguish of a divorced man who recently came to a family agency seeking advice. His ex-wife and her new husband wanted to adopt his two-year-old daughter. In his desire to do what was best for his child he was torn in a painful conflict over what to do.[8]

If the wife is angry at her ex-husband and blames him for the divorce, the children can be used as an instrument with which to control and punish him. In subtle or direct ways she can alienate them from him. Since she is with them for the bulk of the time she can recount stories of the injustices of which he was guilty. Any difficult times she experiences following the divorce also can be attributed to him. In more extreme instances of animosity between the divorced parents she can threaten the children, warning them not to communicate with their father or they will be punished. One divorced father faced with that situation received secret phone calls from his children, made from the homes of the children's friends.

Because he may only have very limited amounts of time to be with them, the divorced father will feel pressured to please his children and retain their good will whenever he is with them. Consequently, he may try to buy their love with goodies and entertainment. He also will be hesitant about disciplining them lest he alienate them from him. They could easily retaliate by behaving in passive, sullen ways when they are with him or by indicating to their mother that they simply don't want to be with him.

His defensive position may produce the humiliating interaction in which he feels compelled to play up to his children. They are boss. They have gained the power over him.

The divorced father who risks alienating his children by disciplining them when he is with them may face a situation where the children, upon return to their mother may detail all of the "horrors" of his behavior. Daddy then stands to be accused of traumatizing the children. On the other hand, if he is lavish with them he may be accused of spoiling them.

The divorced father stands to face a nightmare situation where all the efforts of his married life dissolve in front of him. When I note the devastation in the lives of many divorced men I reflect on the oft-heard refrain of the divorced woman that she is entitled to have all that she can get because she gave up the best years of her life to her ex-husband.

Guidelines For The Divorcing Man

1. Do not enter marriage with the omnipotent belief that it can never happen to you. There is a strong likelihood, according to current divorce statistics, that divorce or separation is an almost fifty-fifty possibility. Therefore, if possible, talk about or even contract the contingencies of that possibility with each other or with a lawyer before marriage.

2. Support your wife's assertiveness during marriage, her educational and occupational development, and anything else that will make her an autonomous, independent person. Then, during divorce, it will make you less vulnerable to guilt regarding her helplessness without you and will make her more secure in terms of her ability to survive using her own resources.

3. Free yourself from notions of victim-victimizer and oppressor-oppressed. Understand that everything that occurs in marriage is the outcome of the interaction, not the responsibility of one person who is labeled the wrongdoer. You are not the heavy because you initiate the separation. If she leaves you, particularly if it is for another man, view it as a growth experience and begin to build a new life. Do not drain your energy in self-accusations or by engaging in futile manipulations to win her back.

4. Free yourself psychologically from guilt and other self-destructive messages once a divorce is in process. Draw a careful line, with the help of a psychologically sophisticated intermediary, between decency or fairness and guilt-motivated, self-punishing behavior.

5. In matters of custody, remember that if you become an occasional father you will find yourself becoming increas-

ingly alienated emotionally from your children. Should your wife remarry you should assume at least an equal share of the custody. Otherwise you are almost certain to lose your children, actually and psychologically, as they begin to attach themselves to their new father.

12. The Hazards
Of Being Male

When a man's self is hidden from everybody else . . . it
seems also to become much hidden even from himself, and it
permits disease and death to gnaw into his substance without
his clear knowledge. Men who are unknown and/or inade-
quately loved often fall ill, or even die, as if suddenly and
without warning . . . If one had direct access to the person's
real self, one would have had many earlier signals that the
present way of life was generating illness.[1]

—Sidney Jourard

Cultural mythology has it that the male is in a favored position. After all, it does appear as if he has more options, more
choices, more power, and greater freedom than the female. If
all of this is in fact true, then he is paying an incredibly high
price for being "top dog" because the facts of his reality are
frightening indeed.

Though there are approximately 105 male babies conceived
for every 100 females,[2] in the population at large there are
today approximately 95 males for every 100 females.[3]

From birth on, the rate of attrition is significantly higher for
the male. There are approximately 115 male fetal deaths for
every 100 female fetal deaths.[4] At nearly every age level, from
birth to death, the male mortality rate is significantly higher.
Specifically, from birth to age one the male death rate is 33
per cent higher. From age 15 to 19, male death rate is more
than 150 per cent higher. From age 20 to 24, male death rate
is over 200 per cent higher and at almost all age levels after
that male death rate is about 100 per cent higher, or *twice as
high as that of the female's!*[5]

The situation is becoming worse. In 1920, the female life
expectancy was only one year higher than that of the male.
Today, the difference is almost eight years and increasing![6]

The gain in life expectancy since 1920 has been greater for women than for men at virtually all ages.

According to a population study at Harvard, if this direction continues, by the turn of the century the elderly would have to take up polygamy because it is predicted that there will be 145 women for every 100 men over the age of sixty-five.[7]

The increasing disparity in longevity cannot simple-mindedly be attributed to some "natural" female biological superiority. Males have larger heart and lung capacities proportionate to their size and a greater capacity for oxygen in the blood which enables them to recover from exhaustion faster. The oldest authenticated age for a human was achieved by a male. That males are showing these dire longevity statistics must be viewed from the perspective of life-styles, stresses, physiological habits, emotional repressions, and sociological pressures.

Being a male is particularly hazardous during boyhood, when supposedly the male is culturally privileged by having greater opportunities for exploration and pleasure. Though the cultural pressures on the boy to behave in traditionally masculine ways is much greater than the pressures on the girl to behave in traditionally female ways ("Tomboy" is cute, "Sissy" is terrible), the growing boy in today's society has precious few live male models who are around enough of the time for him to identify with and to make the passage into adult malehood a smooth or comfortable one.

For the first ten years of his life, the important identification and authority figures around him are mainly females, specifically mother and teacher. (Chances are great that teacher in elementary school will be a woman.) Either Dad works all day and comes home too tired to really get involved, or else the parents are divorced and mother has custody. Consequently, to a great extent, the young boy has to learn to identify himself as a man vicariously by hearing the cultural definition of one from women or through fantasy via television or reading.

The contemporary prevailing trend in parental interaction seems to be one of a dominant mother and a passive father. It appears that increasingly the male parent has faded into the background and turned the reins over to mother. Therefore, even if father is present in the home, he often offers only an elusive, shadowy image with which the young boy can identify.

This situation is aggravated still further for the young son by the fact that on those occasions when father does make an impact it is often in the role of punisher—the heavy. Mother warns her son that if he misbehaves she will tell Dad when he comes home. In the process, therefore, when Dad is not shadowy, he is often a feared and negative identification figure.

The early identification process for the boy is therefore paradoxical and tragic. Pressures are put on him to be "all boy," yet he has to achieve a masculine identification virtually by proxy, via a father who is either uninvolved, often absent, passive when present, or assuming a punitive role.

Despite the liberalized attitude of many contemporary parents who allow boys to behave in the traditionally feminine ways, a recent study indicated that it's still a matter of "pity the poor sissy" for the boy who shows interest in female-type activities.[8]

The director of a gender identity research treatment program at UCLA reported that unlike their "tomboy" counterparts, "sissy" boys are quickly marked for rejection. The boys in this program who are being treated for their effeminate behavior all have suffered harassment. One seven-year-old boy, it was reported, had his shirt torn off by classmates to see if he had female breasts.[9]

Not so surprising is the fact that although girls with "tomboy" patterns would not be excluded from this program they are almost never brought in. Clearly in our culture parents don't seem to get very uptight about their "tomboy" daughters, but they become very disturbed if their sons show "sissy" patterns. This is a destructive cultural paradox regarding the male since research has revealed that both boys and girls identify more closely with mother than with father and that boys have greater difficulty achieving same sex identification.[10]

Early educational experiences for the young boy can also be very painful in many subtle and not-so-subtle ways. In the public schools, the majority of students regarded as problem cases by teachers are boys. A recent study of California school children in schools that permit corporal punishment, indicated that boys were on the receiving end of a spanking by teachers eighteen times more often than girls.[11]

The elementary school setting puts the young boy into more

than his share of painful binds. While there is great peer pressure to act like a boy, the teacher's coveted classroom values are traditionally "feminine" ones. The emphasis is on politeness, neatness, docility, and cleanlinesss, with not much approved room being given for the boy to flex his muscles. Teacher's greatest efforts often go into keeping the boys quiet and in their seats.

A recent study of 12,000 students produced some interesting findings along this line. The researcher correlated masculinity scores of the boys on the California Psychological Inventory with their school grades. She found that the higher the boy scored on the masculine scale, the lower his report card average tended to be.

Of the 277 students with a D or F average, 60 per cent were boys. Of the two boys with the most distinguished scholastic records, one was noted to be markedly effeminate in speech and gesture while the other "gave the strong impression of being more feminine than effeminate." Both boys had very low scores in physical fitness.

The researcher in this study came to the conclusion that "Many schools and academies are dehumanizing and unmanly places. Boys who succeed in them often do so by grossly violating many codes of honor and the norms of boy culture."[12]

The young boy in our culture is placed into countless such dilemmas. He is told he must become a boy but he has to do so with very limited male model availability. He is taught that "real boys" are active and strong but then gets into trouble in school for acting like a "real boy." He is in constant conflict between his own restlessness and the desire to be active and his teacher's demand that he be quiet, submissive, and passive.

It is not surprising then that a study conducted with 1,700 children, the entire kindergarten through second grade population of a midwestern university town, found that boys showed a significantly greater prevalence of behavior symptoms. These included, among others, oddness and bizarre behavior, preoccupation ("in a world of his own"), short attention span, passivity and suggestibility, hyperactivity, negativism, nervousness, poor muscular coordination, distractibility, and inability to relax.

Of fifty-five symptoms, boys showed a significantly greater amount in approximately forty. Girls only showed a significantly greater prevalence in five, which included, "doesn't

know how to have fun," shyness, jealousy over attention paid
to other children, and physical complaints such as stomach-
aches and hypersensitivity ("feelings easily hurt").

The researchers concluded:

> There seems little doubt that not only do boys have more
> symptoms but the connotative sense of most of the symptoms
> commoner in boys represents "badness." Thus it can be con-
> cluded that, at this age level, boys are perceived by female
> teachers as more trouble or "worse" than girls. . . . Thus
> boys must be considered to have a higher rate of disorder
> and to be more "at risk" in our society than girls.[13]

Boys are seen in child guidance clinics at a rate which is
often as high as three times that of the girls. One such major
clinic near a large metropolitan area, serves the entire state of
Michigan and sees a representative sampling of severely disturbed and moderately disturbed children and adolescents. Of
500 children discussed in this reported study, 380 or 76 per
cent were boys. The ratio of boys to girls was slightly higher
than three to one. The ten most common symptoms were poor
academic achievement, behavior problems, reading problems,
aggressiveness, hyperactivity, stealing, oppositional behavior,
poor peer relationships, temper tantrums, and anxiety.[14]

Various reports have suggested that autism, the severest
form of childhood schizophrenia, runs three to four times as
high as for boys.[15] In state and county mental hospital units
for children, boys outnumber girls by approximately 150 per
cent.[16] Under the age of fifteen, males are diagnosed as schizophrenics 42 per cent more frequently than girls.[17]

In light of all of this it is obvious that the "blessings" of
being a young male in our culture are extremely mixed. From
early boyhood on, his emotions are suppressed by others and
therefore repressed by himself. In countless ways he is constantly being conditioned not to express his feelings and needs
openly. Though he too has needs for dependency, he learns
that it is unmasculine to act in a dependent way. It is also
unmasculine to be frightened ("scared"), to want to be held,
stroked, and kissed, to cry, etc. While all of these expressions of self are acceptable in a girl they are incompatible with
the boy's sought after image of being tough and in control.

If he falls and hurts himself he is encouraged to deny his
pain because "big boys don't cry." This attitude carries over

into adolescence when the "hero" of a football or basketball game would be someone who continues to play after he has been injured. Typically, our professional athletes are often drugged and their pains anesthetized as they are thrown back into the fray after non-disabling injuries.

The end result of this is an adult male who tends to disregard, deny, and in general "tune out" body signals of disease and discomfort. He goes to work even when he doesn't feel well and only takes to bed when he is near collapse. Because being ill means being somewhat helpless, passive, and dependent he resists it for much longer than he should.

Because being sick, staying in bed and "pampering" himself are anathema to the masculine image, he may be so deaf to his body signals that he goes from feeling great one day to having a heart attack the next. The signs of impending illness either have been ignored or were never consciously experienced. Consequently, when he finally ends up in the hospital he tends to stay an average of 15 per cent longer than the female.[18]

Other data also bear out the resistance of the male to taking care of himself and to seeking help for body problems. Males make approximately twenty-five per cent fewer visits per year to doctors and dentists than females.[19] Lest it be assumed that this is because males are healthier, the following facts on chronic illnesses leading to death thoroughly dispel this notion.

Men are four to five times more likely to die from bronchitis, emphysema, and asthma than females. Death rates from cardiovascular diseases and cirrhosis of the liver are twice as high. Men die from hypertension approximately 40 per cent more often, from pneumonia and influenza 64 per cent more often, and from arteriosclerosis at a rate of 20 per cent more often.[20]

Tuberculosis hospitals report a male population which is 150 per cent higher and chronic disease hospitals report a male population which is 50 per cent higher.[21]

According to the 1973 statistics of the American Cancer Society, the annual death rate for males from cancer is almost 40 per cent higher.[22] The male rate for specific site cancers such as lung cancer and cancer of the esophagus is even greater than that.

A man in the throes of emotional problems also resists reaching out and seeking help from professionals or friends. Until he finally breaks down altogether he is prone to denying that he even has any problems. He has learned very well to hide and repress his real self, his feelings, and to keep his own counsel. The divorced male is a tragic example of the result of this attitude and "masculine" orientation. For divorced males the death rate is 3.16 times the rate for divorced women.[23] In all institutions, state, county, private, and general hospital in-patient psychiatric services, separated or divorced men outnumber females by 20 per cent. However, in out-patient psychiatric services, separated and divorced females outnumber separated and divorced men by 12 per cent.[24] These figures suggest the greater readiness of the women to ask for help before emotional problems have become so severe as to require institutionalization.

It has been claimed by some feminists that women have more emotional problems and they cite as proof the fact that a greater number of them are in private psychotherapy. However, I believe that going for private therapy actually is a sign of the woman's greater sensitivity and awareness of her feelings, her greater capacity to ask for help and to allow herself to depend on and come close to someone in order to get it. She is possibly also less reluctant to spend money on herself for this purpose than the male and/or in some cases her husband is more willing to spend it on her than on himself. This is suggested by the fact that women outnumber men in private psychiatric facilities by 18 per cent while men are admitted to publicly supported state and county hospitals at a rate which is 20 per cent higher than the female.[25]

The tragedy in the male's resistance to asking for help for emotional problems is that he probably needs it more. Recent studies on stress tolerance suggest that the male has less capacity to cope with stress. A study of one-year-old children, for example, revealed that boys become upset by stress conditions more quickly and require mother's presence near them more in order to cope.[26]

From my own experience as a psychotherapist I would concur with the researcher who concluded, after comparing sex differences in mental health, that "women exhibit greater tolerance of and long range adaptability to stress and frustration . . . [and] women as a group show a greater concern with physical and mental health."[27] Another researcher who has spent more than twenty-five years studying stress, summed it up this way: "Whether you experiment with animals in the laboratory or simply observe everyday life, males invariably go to pieces faster than females. Their endocrine and central nervous systems just don't stand up well under the strain."[28]

Vocational status and employment are another source of hazardous stress in many ways unique to the male. Discussing sex differences in mental health, one researcher pointed out in his monograph that ". . . the positive self-image of the male depends primarily on his success at work. . . . It is very likely that the male needs success in work as a basis for success in love."[29] Psychotherapists have noted that loss of employment, a lowering of job status, or failure in investments often find sexual impotence in its wake.

The man who loses his job may find his identity and self-respect severely threatened. He has learned to value himself on the basis of performance, achievement, and productivity. Many men live in quiet terror of losing their occupational place and struggle desperately to maintain it. In this age of "future shock" every man knows how tenuous his vocational place is and lives in dread of being discarded as obsolete. Retirement, rather than being something to look forward to becomes a fearsome thing. As is well-known, a great proportion of men die shortly after retirement.

Any description of the "joys" of the working life would be incomplete without mentioning that there are about fourteen thousand deaths on the job recorded annually and over two million disabling injuries. A recent study commissioned by the United States Department of Labor indicated that many more serious injuries go uncounted.[30] Men are victims of these accidents, according to government statistics, at a rate which is at least six times higher than women.[31]

The male tragedy is highlighted by the following statistics in criminal and legal matters. He is six times more likely to be arrested on narcotics charges, thirteen times more likely to be arrested for drunkenness, over nine times more likely to be arrested for offenses against children, fourteen times as likely to be arrested for weapons offenses, eleven times more likely to be arrested for gambling, and three times more likely to be arrested for involvement in a motor vehicle accident.[32]

What happens after the arrest? Whereas 83 per cent of total

arrests in 1970 were males, over 95 per cent of those admitted
to state and federal prisons were males.[53] The male is clearly
more likely to be convicted and sentenced to prison.

In 1960, before capital punishment had been temporarily
abolished 21 per cent of those arrested on murder charges
were women. However, only about one per cent (30 out of
3,294) of those executed for murder were female.[54]

Seventeen hundred and twenty felony cases were studied in
1967 to determine the impact personal characteristics of the
offender have on the court's decision. This critical study revealed that, "Women were found to receive much better treatment than male offenders,"—the judges showing "something
of a chivalrous attitude toward women,"—and that "a sub-
stantially higher percentage of women offenders receive sen-
tences involving non-imprisonment than do their male counterparts." Sentencing differences were attributed to the
popular belief that women commit crimes of passion and are
"seldom possessed of pervasive criminal tendencies that more
often characterize male criminals."[55]

The UCLA Law Review recently published a paper on
"Disparities in Criminal Procedure." Using a sampling of 11,-
258 cases from 194 counties in all 50 states the study indicated that "the disparity tends to favor the female, particularly
at the sentencing stage." The study further indicated:

> With regard to pre-trial procedure, male defendants in as-
> sault and larceny cases are much less likely than female de-
> fendants to be released on bail they can afford. . . . The
> federal findings generally tend to show that female defend-
> ants receive more favorable treatment than male defendants.
> . . . With regard to the results of the state criminal process,
> the sample sizes are large enough to say with reasonable
> confidence that the female defendant is more likely than the
> male to be found innocent, and if found guilty is more likely
> to receive a suspended sentence or probation.[56]

While everybody seems to know that men commit significantly more crimes, it is perhaps less well known that they are
also significantly more likely to be the victim. Males are the
victims of aggravated assault 143 per cent more often; 404 per
cent more often the victim of a burglary; 150 per cent more
often the victim of larceny; and 45 per cent more often the
victim of robbery.[57] And according to the 1972 *Uniform*

Crime Reports, men were the victims of murder in approximately 80 per cent of the cases.[38] Although men are arrested for murder six times as often, when it comes to spouse killings which comprise over 10 per cent of all murders, almost half of all of these killings are committed by women.[39]

There is a special hazard to being a male homosexual in our culture. As a recent study pointed out, "The major emphasis of legislation in the field of criminal justice is directed toward the male homosexual, as laws are almost never enforced concerning the female homosexual."[40]

A cursory survey by that researcher of fifteen law enforcement agencies in southern California revealed an apathy toward female homosexuality. Females arrested on charges related to this ranged from 2 to 4 per cent of the total number of arrests for homosexuality. ". . . the Los Angeles Police Department has had a range of 2.9 to 4.3 per cent of a five year period." The researcher concluded that there was almost a ". . . total lack of interest in female homosexuals as a law enforcement problem."[41]

No chapter on the hazards of being male would be complete without a discussion of the suicide statistics. They are perhaps the most telling of all the statistics regarding the "glories" and "joys" of being male. Up to the age of twenty-four the male rate of suicide is over three times as high as the female's. Over the age of sixty-five, the rate is almost five times as high for the male.[42] These statistics do not account for the many automobile accidents leading to death which may actually have been suicides. Men have a twelve times higher ratio of success to failure in suicide attempts in comparison to women. That is, women attempt suicide approximately four times as often as men while men actually *succeed* in killing themselves three times more often.

What may sound like a litany of despair for the male is actually a description of the real crises faced by the male in our culture—crises that will not be remedied simply by the implementation of legislation, but which demand a revolution in male consciousness.

By what perverse logic can the male continue to imagine himself "top dog?" Emotionally repressed, out of touch with his body, alienated and isolated from other men, terrorized by the fear of failure, afraid to ask for help, thrown out at a moment's notice on the occupational junkpile when all he ever knew was how to work, it is perhaps surprising that the suicide statistics are only what they are. Perhaps, however, the male has become an artist in the creation of many hidden ways of killing himself.

Out Of The Harness:
The Free Male

It's the awareness, the full experience . . . of how you are
stuck, that makes you recover, and realize the whole thing is
just a nightmare. . . .[1]

—Frederick S. Perls

The liberated male, in touch with his psychological and
physiological self, will simply not want to disguise and numb
the pressures of a painful harness. He will reject onerous life
situations and ungratifying relationships and environments
that sanctify his role while they deny expression to his being
and to his feelings. He will reject externally imposed, pre-
defined "masculine" roles, not for ideological reasons, but simply because they are painful and self-destructive.

The struggle of the male to learn to listen to and respect his
own intuitive, inner promptings is the greatest challenge of all.
His external social conditioning has been so powerful that it
has all but destroyed his ability to be self-aware. Yet each
denial of his feelings, each faked response, each feigned involvement and each act motivated by guilt or bravado pushes
his destruction further along. It requires a constant self-
awareness and sensitivity to himself in order to avoid the
temptation to be the "nice guy" rather than to do what is real
and true for himself. The male will never give up this role of
accommodating "nice guy" until he has clearly been able to
see how this posture inevitably destroys rather than facilitates.

Male growth will stem from openly avowed, unashamed,
self-oriented motivations. They would include the drive to
preserve himself, to live joyfully, to cherish and ensure his
physical well-being, to get maximal pleasure from his sexuality, to give spontaneous and unashamed expression to his feelings, to openly reveal and share his fantasies, to personalize
rather than objectify his relationships such that distant and

anonymous targets and outlets will not be needed for the expression of anger or the fulfillment of needs vicariously, to remain fluid in his rhythm such that he can be both active and passive with equal comfort and to relate to other men in a sharing, caring way rather than through manipulation and competition. Guilt-oriented "should" behavior will be rejected because it is always at the price of a hidden build-up of resentment and frustration and alienation from others and is, therefore, counterproductive.

The free male will reclaim his total self, coming increasingly in contact with his own unique and individual rhythm rather than living by rigid role casting, imaging, and expectations that result in repetitive, stereotyped responses. He will therefore in certain ways become an unpredictable person because he will not allow his responses to be programmed by external pressure but rather by his inner promptings. He will be sometimes social, sometimes withdrawn, sometimes active, sometimes passive, sometimes sexual, sometimes celibate, sometimes dependent, sometimes independent. In other words, his rhythm and behavior will be variable.

In times when he believes out of a sense of responsibility to meet the needs of another, he would do so only with a constant awareness and vigilance that would allow him to keep a recognition of the separation between his role behavior and his real self.

The free male will constantly reaffirm his right and need to develop and to grow, to be total and fluid, and to have no less than a state of total well-being. He will celebrate all of the many dimensions of himself, his strength and his weakness, his achievements and his failures, his sensuality, his affectionate and loyal response to women and men. He will follow his own personal growth path, making his own stops along the way, and revelling in his unique and ever-developing total personhood.

References

1. In Harness: The Male Condition

1. Abraham Monk, "Factors on the Preparation for Retirement by Middle-Aged Adults," *The Gerontologist*, Winter, 1971, pp. 348–351.
2. Barry Farrell, "You've Come A Long Way, Buddy," *Life*, August 27, 1971, p. 51.

2. Earth Mother Is Dead

1. Albert Martin, "I Am One Man, Hurt," *New York Times*, June 25, 1973, p. 33.
2. Anne Steinmann and David J. Fox, *The Male Dilemma* (New York: Jason Aronson, 1974) p. 140.
3. Walter R. Gove, "The Relationship Between Sex Roles, Marital Status, and Mental Illness," *Social Forces*, September, 1972, pp. 34–44.
4. U.S. Dept. of H.E.W., "Increase in Divorces," *Data from the National Vital Statistics System*, Series 21, No. 20, 1967, p. 14.
5. C. M. Parkes, B. Benjamin, and R. G. Fitzgerald, "Broken Hearts: A Statistical Study of Increased Mortality Among Widowers," *British Medical Journal*, March, 1969, pp. 740–743.
6. Bernard E. Segal, "Suicide and Middle Age," *Sociological Symposium*, No. 3, Fall, 1969.
7. J. Bunch, B. Barraclough, B. Nelson, and P. Sainsbury, "Suicide Following Bereavement of Parents," *Social Psychiatry*, December, 1971, pp. 193–199.
8. Paul C. Glick and Arthur J. Norton, "Frequency, Duration and Probability of Marriage and Divorce," *Journal Marriage and the Family*, 1971, pp. 307–317.

9. Ashley Montagu, as quoted by Myron Brenton in *The American Male* (Greenwich, Conn.: Fawcett Publications, Inc., 1966) p. 199.
10. Steinmann and Fox, *op. cit.*, pp. 121–122.
11. "The Broken Family: Divorce U.S. Style," *Newsweek*, March 12, 1973, pp. 45–57.
12. Ruth Read, "Changing Conceptions of the Maternal Instinct," *Journal of Abnormal and Social Psychology*, Vol. 18, No. 1, 1923, pp. 78–87.
13. Seymour Feshbach and Norma Feshbach, "The Young Aggressors," *Psychology Today*, April, 1973, pp. 90–95.
14. Shana Alexander, "Will Power Change Women?" *Newsweek*, April 1, 1974, p. 30.
15. Susan Edmiston, "Are Psychoanalysis and Feminism Natural Enmies?" *The Village Voice*, June 13, 1974, p. 21.

3. The Wisdom Of The Penis

1. Nikos Kazantzakis, *Zobra The Greek* (New York: Simon and Schuster, 1953) p. 103.
2. Daniel A. Sugarman, "Male Impotence: What every Woman Should Know," *Reader's Digest*, September, 1973, pp. 91–95.
3. Alan J. Cooper, "A Clinical Study of 'Coital Anxiety' in Male Potency Disorders," *Journal of Psychosomatic Research*, Vol. 13, No. 2, 1969, pp. 143–147.
4. Henry David Thoreau, *Walden* (Columbus, Ohio: Charles E. Merrill Publishing Co., 1969) p. 10.
5. M. F. Nimkoff (Ed.), *Comparative Family Systems* (Boston: Houghton Mifflin, 1965) p. 17.
6. Roger N. Johnson, *Aggression in Man and Animals* (Philadelphia: W. B. Saunders Company, 1972) p. 95.
7. *Ibid.*, p. 94.
8. Ralph E. Johnson, "Extramarital Sexual Intercourse: A Methodological Note," *Journal of Marriage and the Family*, May, 1970, pp. 279–282.
9. Harvey E. Kaye, *Male Survival* (New York: Grosset & Dunlap, 1974) p. 77.
10. *L. A. Herald Examiner*, June 27, 1974.
11. "Modern Living," *Time*, February 28, 1969, p. 48.
12. Linda Wolfe, "The Question of Surrogates in Sex Therapy," *New York Magazine*, December 3, 1973, p. 126.

13. "Carnal Knowledge," *Ramparts,* December, 1971, pp. 16–28.
14. Barbara Grizzuti Harrison, "Sexual Chic, Sexual Fascism and Sexual Confusion," *New York Magazine,* April 1, 1974, p. 31.
15. Peter Fisher, *The Gay Mystique* (New York: Stein & Day, 1972) pp. 105–106.

4. FEELINGS: THE REAL MALE TERROR

1. Digby Diehl, "Book Talk: Psychic Echoes of Man on the Moon" (a book review of *Return to Earth* by Buzz Aldrin, Jr., and Wayne Warga), *L.A. Times* Calendar Section, November 25, 1973, p. 61.
2. Mary J. Collier and Eugene L. Gaier, "The Hero in the Preferred Childhood Stories of College Men," *American Image,* Vol. 16, No. 2, 1956, pp. 177–194.

7. THE DESTRUCTION OF THE MALE BODY

1. Pasteur's dying words, reflecting on his long scientific disagreement with Claude Bernard as quoted by Walter McQuade and Ann Aikman in *Stress* (New York: E. P. Dutton & Co., Inc., 1974) p. 18.
2. Clara M. Davis, "Results of Self-Selection of Diets by Young Children," *Canadian Medical Association Journal,* 41, 1939, pp. 257–261.
3. Joseph Brennemann, "Psychologic Aspects of Nutrition in Children," *The Journal of Pediatrics,* August, 1932, p. 170.
4. Morris L. Haimowitz and Natalie Reader Haimowitz (Eds.), *Human Development* (New York: Thomas Y. Crowell Company, 1960) p. 213.
5. Ruth G. Matarazzo, Joseph D. Matarazzo, and George Saslow, "The Relationship Between Medical and Psychiatric Symptoms," *Journal of Abnormal and Social Psychology,* Vol. 62, No. 1, 1961, pp. 55–61.
6. S. M. Weiss, "Psychosomatic Aspects of Symptom Patterns Among Major Surgery Patients," *Journal of Psychosomatic Research,* Vol. 13, No. 1, 1969, pp. 109–112.

7. Eleanor E. Macoby and Carol Nagy Jacklin, "Stress, Activity and Proximity Seeking: Sex Differences in the Year-Old Child," *Child Development*, Vol. 44, 1973, pp. 34–42.

8. Robert M. Stern and J. David Higgins, "Perceived Somatic Reactions to Stress: Sex, Age and Familial Occurrence," *Journal of Psychosomatic Research*, Vol. 13, 1969 pp. 77–82.

9. "The Death of Rudolph Valentino," *New York Times*, August 16, 1926, p. 1.

10. Jack Scott, "It's Not How You Play the Game, But What Pill You Take," *New York Times Magazine*, October 17, 1971, pp. 40–41.

11. Richard M. Kurtz, "Body Image—Male & Female," *Trans-Action*, December, 1968, pp. 25–27.

12. "American Diet Linked to Six Types of Cancer," *Los Angeles Times*, March 26, 1974, Part I, p. 5.

13. "Beef and Bowel Cancer," *Newsweek*, February 18, 1974, pp. 80–83.

14. George Getze "Longevity Diet Will Explode Food Myths, Doctor Predicts," *Los Angeles Times*, December 2, 1973, Part I, p. 3.

15. Joseph V. Brady, "Ulcers in 'Executive Monkeys,'" *Scientific American*, October, 1958, pp. 95–100.

16. Thomas H. Holmes and Minoru Masuda, "Psychosomatic Syndrome," *Psychology Today*, April, 1972, pp. 71–106.

17. David M. Kissin, "Personality Characteristics in Males Conducive to Lung Cancer," *British Journal of Medical Psychology*, Vol. 36, 1963, p. 27.

18. Claus Bahne Bahnson and Marjorie Brooks Bahnson, "Role of the Ego Defenses: Denial and Repression in the Etiology of Malignant Neoplasm," *New York Academy of Sciences Annals*, Vol. 125, May–January, 1965–1966, pp. 827–848.

19. A. H. Buss, *Psychopathology* (New York: John Wiley & Sons, Inc., 1966) p. 414.

20. David Lester, "Voodoo Death: Some New Thoughts on an Old Phenomenon," *American Anthropologist*, Vol. 74, 1972, pp. 386–390.

21. Anne Taylor Fleming, "Up From Slavery—To What?" *Newsweek*, January 21, 1974, pp. 14–15.

8. The Success Trip: A Fantasy Portrait

1. Richard Brooks and James Poe, screenplay of *Cat on a Hot Tin Roof* by Tennessee Williams, an Avon Production for Metro-Goldwyn-Mayer, 1959.

9. The Lost Art Of Buddyship

1. Stan Levine, "One Man's Experience," *MS*, February, 1973, p. 14.

10. Marriage: Guilt By Association

1. Nathan W. Ackerman in Harold Hart (Ed.), *Marriage: For and Against* (New York: Hart Publishing Co., Inc., 1972) p. 13.
2. William J. Lederer in Harold Hart (Ed.), *Marriage: For and Against, Ibid.*, p. 135.
3. Gene Lester and David Lester, *Suicide: The Gamble With Death* (Englewood Cliffs, New Jersey: Prentice-Hall, 1971) p. 67.
4. Dee G. Applezweig, "Childhood and Mental Health: The Influence of the Father in the Family Setting," *Merrill-Palmer Quarterly*, April, 1971, p. 71.
5. Helene S. Arnstein, "The Crisis of Becoming a Father," *Sexual Behavior*, April, 1972, pp. 42–47.
6. *Ibid.*, p. 47.
7. C. Nydegger, "The Older the Father: Late Is Great," *Psychology Today*, April, 1974, pp. 26–28.

11. Divorce: The Penalties For Leaving

1. George R. Bach and Herb Goldberg, *Creative Aggression* (Garden City, New York: Doubleday & Co., 1974).
2. Paul C. Glick and Arthur J. Morton, "Frequency, Duration and Probability of Marriage and Divorce," *Journal of Marriage and the Family*, May, 1971, p. 310.
3. Peter Arnett, "New Ordeal for Ex-POW—The Heartbreak of Divorce," *Los Angeles Times*, April 22, 1973, Part I, p. 1.

4. Former Calif. Civ. Code #139, cited in Honorable William P. Hogoboom, "The California Family Law Act of 1970: 18 Months Experience," *Missouri Bar Journal*, 27, 1971, pp. 584–589.
5. *Ibid.*, p. 586.
6. James Lincoln Collier, "Time to Give Divorced Men a Break," *Reader's Digest*, February, 1970, p. 66.
7. William J. Goode, *After Divorce* (New York: The Free Press, 1956) pp. 298, 336.
8. Anne C. Schwartz, "Reflections on Divorce and Remarriage," *Social Casework*, April, 1968, p. 214.

12. THE HAZARDS OF BEING MALE

1. Sidney Jourard, *The Transparent Self* (revised edition) (Princeton, N.J.: Van Nostrand Co.) 1971, p. 40.
2. U.S. Bureau of the Census, *Statistical Abstracts of the United States, 1973* (Washington, D.C.: Government Printing Office, 1973) p. 52.
3. U.S. Bureau of the Census, based on *U.S. Census of Population, 1950; 1960; 1970; General Population Characteristics*, final report PC (1)-BI, *United States Summary*. This information is cited by the U.S. Bureau of the Census in *Statistical Abstracts of the United States, 1972* (Washington, D.C.: Government Printing Office, 1972) p. 24.
4. U.S. National Center for Health Statistics, *Vital Statistics for the United States, 1967*, Mortality, Part A (Washington, D.C.: Government Printing Office, Vol. II, 1969) pp. 3–5.
5. U.S. National Center for Health Statistics, *Vital Statistics for the United States*, cited in *Statistical Abstracts of the United States, 1973, op. cit.*, pp. 57–58.
6. *Ibid.*
7. *Los Angeles Times*, February 10, 1974, Part I, p. 4.
8. "King of the Sandbox," *Human Behavior*, June, 1973, p. 37.
9. "Girlish Boys" *Time*, November 26, 1973, p. 33.
10. David B. Lynn, "The Process of Learning Parental and Sex-Role Identification," in Dirk L. Schaeffer (Ed.), *Sex Differences in Personality: Readings* (Belmont, Calif., Wadsworth Publishing Co., 1971) pp. 41–49.

11. *Los Angeles Times,* February 8, 1974, Part I, p. 3.
12. Patricia Sexton, "How the American Boy is Feminized," *Psychology Today,* January, 1970, pp. 23–29; 66–67.
13. John S. Werry and Herbert C. Quarry, "The Prevalence of Behavior Symptoms in Younger Elementary School Children," *American Journal of Orthopsychiatry,* January, 1971, pp. 136–143.
14. Charles R. Shaw, *The Psychiatric Disorders of Childhood* (New York: Appleton-Century Crofts, 1966) p. 64.
15. L. Eisenberg and L. Kanner, "Early Infantile Autism," *American Journal of Orthopsychiatry,* 26, 1956, pp. 55–65.
    C. N. Rutt and D. R. Offord, "Prenatal and Perinatal Complications in Childhood Schizophrenics and Their Siblings," *The Journal of Nervous and Mental Disease,* 152, Vol. 5, 1971, pp. 324–331.
16. U.S. Public Health Service, *Statistical Note 72:* "Age, Sex and Diagnostic Conditions of Resident Patients in State and County Mental Hospitals—United States—1961–1970," December, 1972, p. 2.
17. "Schizophrenics in County and State Mental Hospitals by Sex and Age," H.E.W., N.I.M.H., Survey and Reports Section, 1970.
18. U.S. Public Health Service information and published data in *Statistical Abstracts of the United States, 1972* (Washington, D.C.: Government Printing Office, 1972) p. 74.
19. *Ibid.,* p. 69.
20. U.S. Public Health Service information cited in *Associated Press Almanic,* 1973, p. 290.
21. Bureau of the Census, *U.S. Census of Population, 1960,* Vol. II, part PC(2)-8A, cited in U.S. Public Health Service information and unpublished data, *Statistical Abstracts of the United States, 1972* (Washington, D.C.: Government Printing Office, 1972) p. 43.
22. American Cancer Society data cited in *Associated Press Almanac, op. cit.,* p. 292.
23. U.S. Public Health Service, "Increases in Divorce," (Data from the *National Vital Statistics System*) Series 21, No. 20, 1967, p. 14.
24. U.S. Public Health Service, *Statistical Note 81.* "Differen-

tial Utilization of Psychiatric Facilities by Men and Women—United States—1970," June, 1973, p. 9.

25. *Ibid.*
26. E. E. Macoby and C. N. Jacklin, "Stress, Activity and Proximity Seeking Sex Differences in the Year-Old Child," *Child Development,* Vol. 44, 1, 1973, pp. 34–42.
27. J. E. Gari, "Sex Differences in Mental Health," *Genetic Psychological Monographs,* Vol. 81, 1970, pp. 123–142.
28. Ruth Winter, "Biological Superiority—Female or Male," *Science Digest,* August, 1971, p. 50.
29. Gari, *op. cit.,* p. 128.
30. Jerome B. Gordon, *et al., Industrial Safety Statistics: A Re-examination; A Critical Report Prepared for the Department of Labor* (New York: Praeger Publishers, 1971).
31. U.S. National Center for Health Statistics, *Health Statistics from the U.S. National Health Survey; Vital and Health Statistics,* Series 10, No. 72 and unpublished data cited in *Statistical Abstracts of the United States, 1973, op. cit.,* p. 81.
32. Federal Bureau of Investigation, *Uniform Crime Reports for the United States, 1970,* cited in *Statistical Abstracts of the United States, 1972, op. cit.,* p. 150.
33. *Ibid.,* and U.S. Bureau of Prisons, *National Prisons Statistics Bulletin,* No. 47, cited in *ibid.,* p. 160.
34. *Ibid.,* p. 164.
35. Mark C. Clements, "Sex and Sentencing," *Southwestern Law Journal,* Vol. 26, 1972, pp. 890–904.
36. S. S. Nagel, "Disparities in Criminal Procedure," *U.C.L.A. Law Review,* Vol. 14, 1967, pp. 1272–1305.
37. Executive Office of the President, The President's Commission on Law Enforcement and Administration of Justice, *The Challenge of Crime in a Free Society, 1967,* cited in *Statistical Abstracts of the United States, 1972, op. cit.,* p. 145.
38. Federal Bureau of Investigation, "Crime in the United States," *Uniform Crime Reports* (Washington, D.C.: Government Printing Office, August 8, 1973) p. 6.
39. *Ibid.,* pp. 8–9.
40. Harold K. Becker, "A Phenomenological Inquiry into the Etiology of Female Homosexuality," *Journal of Human Relations,* Vol. 17, 1969, pp. 570–579.

41. *Ibid.*, p. 573.
42. U.S. National Center for Health Statistics, unpublished data cited in *Statistical Abstracts of the United States, 1973, op. cit.*, p. 63.

OUT OF THE HARNESS: THE FREE MALE

1. Frederick S. Perls, *Gestalt Therapy Verbatim* (California: Real People Press, 1969) p. 40.

Index